T0185587

Religion and Coping
in
Mental Health Care

INTERNATIONAL SERIES
IN THE PSYCHOLOGY OF RELIGION

14

Edited by

J.A. Belzen

Religion and Coping
in
Mental Health Care

Joseph Pieper
&
Marinus van Uden

Amsterdam - New York, NY 2005

The paper on which this book is printed meets the requirements of "ISO 9706: 1994, Information and documentation - Paper for documents - Requirements for permanence".

ISBN: 90-420-1997-2
Editions Rodopi B.V., Amsterdam - New York, NY 2005
Printed in The Netherlands

UTP-KATERN 26

Religion and Coping in Mental Health Care

The UTP-Katernen is a Series of Scientific Publications in the Domains of Theology, Pastoral Care, Society and Culture. This series is supported by the Edmond Beel Stichting.

CONTENTS

ACKNOWLEDGEMENTS

For the realisation of this volume support was necessary. We are grateful to the Edmond Beel Stichting who sponsored this project. Our gratitude is also owed to the UTP-Katernen Series for their editorial hospitality.

We want to thank as well prof.dr. Hans Alma, University for Humanistics, Utrecht and Leiden University, the Netherlands, for her contribution to the chapters 6 and 7. We also thank Ad van Heeswijk, C. Psychol., Clinical Psychologist, Psychological Therapies NHS Service, Isle of Wight, Great Britain, for his help in the translation of many of the texts included in this volume. Thanks finally to Olaf van Amelsvoort for making the text camera ready.

Chapter 1:
Mental Health and Religion. A Complex Relationship.

First published as:
Pieper, J.Z.T. & Uden, van M.H.F. (1997) Mental Health and Religion. A Complex Relationship. *Archiv für Religionspsychologie 22*, 219-236.

Chapter 2:
Religion in Mental Health Care: Patients' Views.

First published as:
Pieper, J.Z.T & Uden, van M.H.F. (1996) Religion in Mental Health Care: Patients' Views. In: Verhagen, P.J. & Glas, G. (eds.) *Psyche and Faith. Beyond Professionalism.* Zoetermeer: Boekencentrum, 69-83.

Chapter 3:
Religion in Mental Health Care: Psychotherapists' Views.

First published as:
Uden, van M.H.F. & Pieper, J.Z.T. (2000) Religion in Mental Health Care: Psychotherapists' Views. *Archiv für Religionspsychologie 23,* 264-277.

Chapter 4:
Psychotherapy and Religious Problems.
Illustration by Means of a Case History.

First published as:
Uden, van M.H.F. (2000) Psychotherapy and Religious Problems. *Archiv für Religionspsychologie 23*, 243-252.

Chapter 5:
Religious Coping in Two Samples of Psychiatric Inpatients.

Combination of two publications:
Pieper, J.Z.T. (2003) Religious Resources of Psychiatric Inpatients. *Archiv für Religionspsychologie 25*, 142-154.
Pieper, J.Z.T. (2004) Religious Coping in Highly Religious Psychiatric Inpatients. *Mental Health, Religion and Culture 7/4*, 349-363.

Chapter 6:
"When I Find Myself in Times of Trouble…".
Pargament's Religious Coping Scales in the Netherlands.

First published as:
Alma, H.A., Pieper, J.Z.T. & Uden, van M.H.F. (2003) "When I Find Myself in Times of Trouble…". Pargament's Religious Coping Scales in the Netherlands. *Archiv für Religionspsychologie 24*, 64-74.

Chapter 7:
"Bridge over Troubled Water".
Further Results Regarding The Receptive Coping Scale.

First published as:
Uden, van M.H.F., Pieper, J.Z.T. & Alma, H.A. (2004) "Bridge over Troubled Water". Further Results Regarding The Receptive Coping Scale. *Journal of Empirical Theology 17*, 101-114.

Chapter 8:
Clinical Psychology of Religion. A Training Model.

First published as:
Uden, van M.H.F. & Pieper, J.Z.T. (2003) Clinical Psychology of Religion. A Training Model. *Archiv für Religionspsychologie 25*, 155-164.

INTRODUCTION

We will start this introduction by substantiating this volume's basic assumption: the necessity of attention to faith and worldview in mental health care. We will do this by making connections with the results of research in the area of 'religious coping', carried out in the United States. After this, we will briefly indicate the findings of our own research in this area in the Netherlands. Our research was focused, on the one hand, on the position that, according to clients, faith and worldview have in their coping with their mental health problems; on the other hand, on the position that therapists assign to this dimension in the treatment process. In the subsequent chapters of this volume, these data will be further elaborated. We will continue this introduction with some conclusions about the research results' significance for mental health care, and we will finish with a preview of the chapters of this volume.

1. Religious coping

In the psychology of religion, the study of the relationship between religion and mental health has always been a main theme. Already at the discipline's inception at the end of the nineteenth century, James (1994/1902) explored the boundaries between, on the one hand, profound religious and mystical experiences and, on the other hand, psychopathology, whilst Leuba (1896) and Starbuck (1899) were concerned with the significance of conversion experiences for the converts' mental health. In Chapter 1 of this volume we will consider at length the complex relationship that exists between the phenomena of religion and mental health. In the last few decades, this relationship has been studied in particular within the 'religious coping' paradigm, that has been formulated most comprehensively by the American psychologist of religion Kenneth Pargament (1997; see also Harrison 2001). In this line of research, a bridge is being built from theory to the practice of physical and mental health care. Many studies are concerned with the significance of religion for coping with physical and mental health problems in people admitted to a general or psychiatric hospital. Within this approach, religion is portrayed as a positive force in conquering physical and mental adversities.

Let us first consider the 'coping' aspect of 'religious coping'. Research on coping has flourished in particular with the rise of cognitive psychology, within which coping processes are seen as a form of information processing, in which the individual is not being directed by structural personality characteristics, but engages in a dynamic interaction with the environment. Lazarus & Folkman (1984) have developed the most elaborate theory. They define 'stress' as follows, "Psychological stress is a particular relationship between person and environment that is appraised by the person as taxing or exceeding his/her resources and endangering his/her well-being". Hence, stress is not an automatic response of the individual to a stimulus, but is the consequence of a process in which the cognitive appraisal and assessment of the stressor play an important role. It will be obvious that people differ in the extent to which they experience stress with the same stressor. This 'cognitive appraisal' is a mental process in which a differentiation can be made between 'primary appraisal' and 'secondary appraisal'. 'Primary appraisal' refers to the question whether a situation or event counts as a threat to the individual's well-being. 'Secondary appraisal', on the other hand, relates to the assessment of the resources that a person has for meeting the requirements of the situation or event. These resources are diverse: material (money, shelter, food, transport), physical (health, vitality), psychological (insight, motivation, knowledge, emotional skills), social (the extent of social support, social networks) and religious (e.g. closeness to God, embeddedness in a religious community).

After these cognitive appraisals, the individual makes efforts to manage the situation, i.e. the actual coping. Coping is "a cognitive and behavioral effort to master, tolerate, or reduce external and internal demands and conflicts among them" (Folkman & Lazarus 1980). According to Folkman & Lazarus (1980), a differentiation has to be made between two forms of coping, *viz.* 'emotion-focused' coping (refers to control of the emotional response to the stressor) and 'problem-focused' coping (aiming at solving the problem by modifying the situation or by changing one's own behaviour). Some also use here the terms 'palliative and instrumental coping'. Although problem-focused coping (e.g. gathering information or seeking help) used to be seen as the more effective form of coping, the assumption nowadays is that the effectiveness of coping behaviour largely depends on the possibility of taking action in a certain situation. As such, effective coping in an unchangeable situation means that no problem-solving behaviour will take place, but that emotion regulating work will be done. In this context, Pargament (1997) referred to the following prayer, "God, grant me serenity to accept the things I cannot change, courage to change the things I can, and wisdom to know the difference". The elderly in particular use emotion regulating strategies, because they have fewer of the physical, social and economic resources that are necessary for action-oriented coping, because they more often consider situations to be unchangeable, and because they are more often confronted with experiences of loss (loss of work, health, friends and loved ones). An important question regarding these coping activities is: why do they arise, what are their fundamental motivations? This concerns the functions of coping behaviour. A very important motive is, of course, the need to solve the problem, but in emotion-focused coping the point is also the maintenance of our psychological equilibrium. In this context, we want to mention three motives: the need for control regarding the arrangement of one's own life; the need for meaningmaking; and the need for maintaining or enhancing one's sense of self-respect. Finally, much attention is paid in the coping literature to the effects of the coping process, at the physical, the psychosocial and the existential levels.

Let us now turn to the religious aspect of religious coping. Here, we rely in particular on Pargament's (1997) book *The Psychology of Religion and Coping*. According to this investigator, religious coping focuses on 'the search for significance'. In coping too the intentionality of human action finds expression. This relates to maximising central values, and not to a rapid reduction of the tensions connected with stress. Coping not only results in the removal of the stressor, but also in the coper's growth (accumulation of significance). In the coping process, this 'search for significance' can be filled in in two ways: either old values will be retained and emphasised ('conservation of significance'), or new values will emerge ('transformation of significance'). Often, religious coping will only occur where non-religious coping fails. In particular in situations of loss of life, health or relational embeddedness, religious coping often will be one of the last remaining emotion-focused coping strategies. Are there situations that are pre-eminently managed in a religious way? This usually refers to profoundly influential life events, to boundary situations for which there are no satisfactory inner-worldly explanations. Also situations that injure the sense of justice often lead to religious emotion management. Within religious coping, a differentiation can be made between individual and social/institutional religious coping, i.e. on the one hand, private religious acts or, on the other hand, church attendance or asking a pastor for help (institutional). In the latter case, the religious dimension is closely linked with obtaining social support. Social support is a very important variable in religious coping research. To illustrate the extent of the occurrence of religious coping, we refer to an investigation by Tepper *et al.* (2001) about the degree to which people with long-standing psychological complaints used religious coping behaviour. 80% of their Los Angeles respondents indicated that their faith or their devotional activities contributed to their coping with their symptoms, difficulties and frustrations.

Research on religious coping has also been considering the effects of religious coping on the respondents' physical, psychological, social and spiritual well-being. In this way, it connects with a research line that exists already since a long time in the psychology of religion, regarding the link between religion and mental health. Research has been carried out into the effects of religious coping upon origin and course of depression in the elderly; psychiatric patients' managing of psychosocial problems; dealing with being a victim of the Oklahoma bombing; caring for a chronically ill child; dealing with losing a relative through suicide; dealing with a renal transplant; students' dealing with relational problems; dealing with cancer; managing the loss of a child through cot death; dealing with parents' divorce; loss of employment; coming to terms with the Gulf War; etc. In general, the effects are positive. Recent reviews (Harrison 2001; Matthews *et al.* 1998) conclude that the greater part of published empirical data shows that religious coping has a favourable influence on dealing with mental and physical illness. Daaleman has summarised the possibilities of religion as follows: "through social integration and support; through the establishment of personal relationships with a divine order; through the provision of systems of meaning and existential coherence, and through the promotion of more specific patterns of religious organization and personal lifestyle" (Daaleman 1999, 220). In keeping with this, this predominantly American research argues that neglecting faith and religion in physical and mental health care, leaves an important source of health promotion unused.

Finally, we have to note that the coping paradigm emphasises that religion's positive effects on well-being usually only occur when the individual's general religiosity can be transformed into concrete religious coping activities with respect to the stressor. Religious coping mediates between general religiosity and well-being. This is the so-called 'stress-buffering model', which contrasts with the 'main-effect model' in which religion, broadly speaking, results in an existence with more well-being, also when separate from its influence on the coping process.

2. Religious coping in Dutch mental health care

The above mentioned positive findings originate mainly from research in the United States. It is a well-known fact that the American population is more religious than the population in the more secularised Netherlands. Moreover, much research is carried out by researchers with a manifestly positive regard for, in particular, the Jewish-Christian tradition. This implies that their findings cannot be automatically transposed to the Netherlands (see chapters 6 and 7 in this volume). We will now briefly describe some important results from our own research in the past ten years, which we carried out among clients and therapists in community and residential mental health care in the Netherlands (this research is reported comprehensively in chapters 2, 3 and 5 in this volume). When we survey the client data, it is clear that for 39% (community) to 54% (residential) of people with mental health problems faith and worldview contribute positively to their coping with their problems. In particular for hospitalised elderly patients, faith and worldview are an important source of coping with regard to their psychosocial problems. We have drawn here the following conclusion: "Patients who are hospitalised in institutions experience their life situation as relatively unchangeable. They lack coping resources focused at problem-solving. For that reason, they revert to coping resources focused at emotionally managing their problems. One of the most important emotion-focused coping resources is religion" (Pieper & Van Uden 2001, 39). However, faith and worldview can also have a negative influence. This was mentioned by 36% of community and 16% of residential patients.

The above data show that also in the Dutch situation, attention to faith and worldview for many patients can contribute to an improvement of their life situation. Positive influences can be supported and negative influences can be tempered. In order for faith and worldview to attain a place in the treatment process, psychotherapists will have to have knowledge of and concern for faith and worldview. Our 1996 research among therapists (see chapter 3 in this volume) can provide some insight regarding this issue. On the subject of their faith/worldview background, we can infer the following. Compared to the average Dutch citizen, therapists believe less in God, attend church less often, believe less in the existence of a transcendent reality, and less often have religious experiences. With respect to the relationship between faith/worldview and psychosocial problems, therapists think that such a relationship exists in only about 18% of clients. They see equally often positive and negative influences of faith/worldview on the problems. Negative influence is, according to the therapists, particularly connected with guilt problems, sexual problems and depression. Positive influence is, according to them, in particular connected with the healthy effects of religious rituals upon the processing of experiences of loss. When faith and worldview aspects are playing a role, most therapists state that they will address them. At the same time, a majority (two thirds) of them thinks that they do not have sufficient skills to treat these aspects adequately; connected with this, 46% indicate a need for further training. They hardly use specific religious therapeutic techniques. Contacts with clergy/chaplaincy are sparse; through-referrals to them occur in only 1% of cases. There is ambivalence regarding enhancement of these contacts.

Clients provided us with additional data. How satisfied are they with the degree to which and the way in which therapists treated the faith and worldview aspects of their problems? Two-thirds of former clients show satisfaction in their response to the question, "Did the Riagg [community mental health agency] offer sufficient opportunity to address the faith/worldview aspects of your problems?". One client states, "My therapist was open to my worldview and respected me regarding this issue. She herself didn't have the same belief as I did, and she frankly admitted that she didn't know whether my thinking in this respect was right or wrong. But she did use my worldview in her therapy with me!" About 60% of respondents is satisfied in response to the question, "Does the therapist usually understand what you mean when talking about faith/worldview questions?" Yet, at the same time, only one third is satisfied with the way in which their treatment connected with the faith/worldview aspects of their problems. In one client's words, "I could tell how I dealt with my faith problems. But I didn't get an answer. She herself didn't know faith, much to my regret." It appears that therapists are able and willing to listen with regard to faith and worldview, but that in their treatments they find it harder to take adequate initiatives in this area.

3. Conclusions

To start with, based on the above we can draw a number of conclusions about the significance of faith and worldview for coping with psychosocial problems. Coping research in the United States indicates primarily a positive effect of faith and worldview, and hence recommends that structurally space is secured to faith and worldview in treatment. Our own research among community and residential patients in the Netherlands also showed that faith and worldview support between 39% (community) and 54% (residential) of them in emotionally coping with their problems. However, we also found faith to have a negative influence, in particular in community patients. This means that therapists should have sufficient knowledge of and concern with faith and worldview. However, many therapists feel that they lack skills in this area, and almost half of them indicate a need for additional training. The clients' opinions point in the same direction: therapists are able and willing to listen to their faith/worldview narratives, but lack the skills for making adequate treatment interventions in this area. Clients often also indicate the therapists' inadequate knowledge regarding religious beliefs and practices (the case study in chapter 4 will show the very complexity of treatment in this area).

All these conclusions taken together justify the recommendation that the faith/worldview dimension should get a more prominent place in treatment than is presently the case, in order to guarantee quality treatment for clients having faith/worldview aspects in their problems. To this end, additional training for professionals in mental health care is a necessary interim step. In our research among therapists, it became manifest that about half of them indicated a wish for more training in the area of faith and worldview. As a start, we have begun to develop, and to pilot in several places, a so called problem-oriented training module in "Clinical Psychology of Religion". We will present this training model in the final chapter (chapter 8) of this volume.

4. Preview

Finally, we will present a synopsis of the following chapters in this volume.

In the first chapter we give an overview of the complex relationship between mental health and religion. We start with a discussion of the concept of mental health. Next we present five ways in which mental health and religion are connected: religion as therapy, suppression of deviant behaviour by religious socialization, religion as a haven, religion as an expression of mental disorder and religion as a hazard to mental health. These different connections will be illustrated by several cases from the literature and clinical work. Briefly formulated, religion can hinder as well as promote mental health. The chapter ends with a critical methodological discussion on how to explain some of these contradictory connections.

Because of the lack of empirical evidence, in 1992 we started a research project among community mental health care patients in the Netherlands, the results of which are presented in chapter 2. How do patients evaluate their treatment? In order to get an answer, we questioned about 425 former clients of the Heerlen Riagg (a community mental health agency situated in a mainly Roman Catholic region in the Netherlands) and about 330 former clients of the Zwolle Riagg (situated in a highly Protestant region in the Netherlands). The questions addressed three main areas. Firstly, we asked about the ways in which religion and worldview are related to mental health problems: is there any relation, and if so, is this a positive or a negative one? Secondly, we asked about the ways in which therapists had reacted to these religious and worldview dimensions: had they been dealt with as relevant to therapy or had they been avoided? Thirdly, we asked some questions about the former clients' wishes and needs regarding the roles religious and worldview dimensions should play in therapy.

In the third chapter we concentrate on the results from an investigation among Riagg therapists, but we also refer to some results obtained from Gliagg therapists (therapists working in a community mental health agency with a more explicit religious signature). This is done in order to clarify in which ways Riagg therapists differ from Gliagg therapists in managing religious aspects of their clients' problems. The investigation started with an overview of the religious backgrounds and religious practices of the therapists. Some equations with average Dutch citizens are made. The next part of the study deals with psychotherapists' perceptions of religious issues connected with psychosocial problems. How often in their opinion is there a relationship, and what kind of relationship is at issue? The third part of the study considers the way in which psychotherapists treat these religious issues. Do they attend to them and what kinds of religious interventions are used? Special attention is given to the amount of contacts with clergy/chaplaincy. We conclude that religion should be given a more pronounced place in general mental health care and that Riagg psychotherapists in particular should become better equipped to deal with religious issues.

In the next chapter (chapter 4) the case history of a patient with an obsessive-compulsive disorder is presented. We show how important it is to look at the religious frame of reference of a patient and how this can be managed in psychotherapeutic treatment. The case is positioned within the theoretical perspective of symbolic interactionism. Through this case we want to show how complex the role of religion is in the individual's psyche. Even in an a-religious (often even anti-religious) psychotherapeutic approach like cognitive behaviour therapy, attention paid to religion and meaning can be of great importance. Challenging negative religious cognitions and offering more positive ones leads to psychotherapeutic progress. In general, the training of counsellors and psychotherapists leaves hardly any room for paying attention to this dimension of existence.

Some results of a study among two samples of psychiatric patients in mental hospitals in the Netherlands are presented in chapter 5. We focus on the following issues:
- the religious and spiritual beliefs and activities of the inpatients;
- their religious coping activities, measured using Pargament's three coping styles and a positive religious coping scale;
- the influence of religious coping on psychological and existential well-being;
- the predictive value of general religiousness, as compared with religious coping activities, regarding psychological and existential well-being.

For these populations of inpatients, religion had a positive influence on their ways of dealing with problems; religious coping was positively correlated with existential and psychological well-being. General religiousness as well as religious coping were positively correlated with existential well-being, whereas psychological well-being primarily was predicted by positive religious coping. We discuss the results in the context of theoretical notions of religious coping, addressing in particular the positive influence of religious beliefs, relying on God, religious activities and religious social support in times of psychological and existential crisis.

The chapter "When I find myself in times of trouble..." (chapter 6) reports on our attempts to use Pargament's three religious problem-solving styles in the Netherlands, on the problems we have met and on the alternative scale we have tried to develop: the Receptivity Scale. The main problem with Pargament's threefold conceptualisation of religious coping (self-directing, deferring and collaborative) is the underlying view of an active, personal God. This ignores the idea of a more impersonal God, which is probably more common in the secularised Netherlands. The Receptivity Scale does justice to this more impersonal view of God. Furthermore, the scale takes into account that people are not always directly focused on the solution of problems, either with or without God. A receptive attitude might allow them to be open to what they cannot control. Confronted with a problematic situation, people can be open to what might be in store for them. The scale we present consists of three items in which no reference is made to a specific interpretation of a transcendent reality. The items are about trust, finding deeper meaning, about receptivity, and enlightenment. The scale yielded some interesting results, but we came to the conclusion that it was too brief and that more items should be added.

The chapter "Bridge over troubled water" (chapter 7) presents a more definitive version of our so-called Receptivity Scale. This version was administered to two populations in Belgium and two in the Netherlands. We examine the precise meaning of this scale by comparing the respondents' scores on the scale with their scores on other measures of religiosity and other psychological measures. We also compare the scores of theology students with the scores of psychology students on the scale. In this way, we obtain more insight in the validity of the scale. In our investigation among 77 psychology students and 36 theology students, we relate the results of our Receptivity Scale to the results of Pargament's coping scales, to a Basic Trust Scale and to an Anxiety Scale. Our research showed that the Receptivity Scale consisted of two subscales: one referring indirectly to an agent who helps coping with problems, and another one referring to an attitude of trust without feeling helped by an agent. 'Receptive-agent' relates positively to religiosity and to the deferring and collaborative coping styles in which the person feels helped by God. It is negatively related to the self-directing scale. 'Receptive-no agent', however, is not significantly related to any of the scales mentioned. It is positively related to basic trust and to commitment to the transcendent. We conclude that this coping style is less clearly religious in the traditional sense of a belief in God than 'receptive-agent', but still it differs from basic trust in its positive relationship with a conception of transcendence. We come to the conclusion that between the basic attitudes of trust on the one hand and trust in a personal God on the other hand, there are different degrees of relating to the transcendent in times of trouble. 'Receptive-agent' comes closer to belief in God; 'receptive-no agent' comes closer to, but is not the same as, basic trust in general.

In the final chapter (chapter 8) we present part of a course in "Clinical Psychology of Religion" that has been developed in the Netherlands with the aim of introducing mental health professionals into the field of the clinical psychology of religion. Clinical psychology of religion aims at applying insights from the general psychology of religion to the field of clinical psychology. Clinical psychology of religion can be defined as that part of the psychology of religion that deals with the relationship between religion, worldview and mental health. Like the clinical psychologist, the clinical psychologist of religion deals with psychological assessment and psychotherapy, but concentrates on the role religion or worldview play in mental health problems. This course uses a special teaching method: Problem Oriented Education. In our research we have found that there is substantial need among psychotherapists to become better equipped in this area. Hence, this course could fill a gap.

In summary

This volume consists of eight previously published papers on the topics of religion, coping, and mental health care. The papers cover a broad territory: the complex relationships between religion and mental health, surveys that present the views of therapists and patients about the interface between religion and mental health, a case study of a religious patient struggling with psychological problems, empirical studies of religious coping among various groups, and a method for teaching the clinical psychology of religion. Although the papers are diverse, they are unified by several themes. First, the papers convey a balanced approach to religion and psychology. They address the potentially positive and negative contributions religion can make to health and well-being. Second, several of the papers focus on the role of religious coping among patients in the Netherlands. This focus is noteworthy, since the large majority of this kind of theory and research has been limited to the United States. Third, they underscore the value of a cross-cultural approach to the field. The surveys point to the importance of religious/worldview perspectives to many patients (and therapists) in the Netherlands, even though Dutch culture is more secularised than the United States. However, the papers also suggest that the manifestation of these religious/worldview perspectives may take different shape in the Netherlands. For example, we identify another form of religious coping based on the notion of "receptiveness" that does not rest on beliefs in a personally active God. Fourth, the papers have clinical relevance. The case history of the obsessive-compulsive patient contains an example of the way in which religious resources can be accessed to counteract dysfunctional behaviours.

References

Daaleman, T.P. (1999) Belief and Subjective Well-being in Outpatients. *Journal of Religion and Health 38*, 219-227.

Folkman, S. & Lazarus, R.S. (1980) An Analysis of Coping in a Middle-aged Community Sample. *Journal of Health and Social Behaviour 21*, 219-239.

James, W. (1902) *The Varieties of Religious Experience. A Study in Human Nature*. New York: Modern Library Press, 1994 (original 1902).

Harrison, M.O. (2001) The Epidemiology of Religious Coping. A Review of Recent Literature. *International Review of Psychiatry 13*, 86-96.

Lazarus, R.S. & Folkman, S. (1984) *Stress, Appraisal, and Coping*. New York: Springer.

Leuba, J.H. (1896) A Study in the Psychology of Religious Phenomena. *American Journal of Psychology 7*, 309-385.

Matthews, D.A., McCullough, M.E., Larson, D.B., Koenig, H.G., Swyers, J.P. & Greenwold Milano, M. (1998) Religious Commitment and Health Status. A Review of the Research and Implications for Family Medicine. *Archive for Family and Medicine 7*, 118-124.

Pargament, K.I. (1997) *The Psychology of Religion and Coping. Theory, Research, Practice*. New York: The Guilford Press.

Pieper, J.Z.T. & Uden, van M.H.F. (2001) *Geestelijke verzorging op De Fontein. Onderzoek onder cliënten van De Fontein naar hun geloof/levensbeschouwing en naar hun behoefte aan geestelijke verzorging [Pastoral Care at De Fontein. Research among Clients of De Fontein regarding their Faith/Worldview and their Need of Pastoral Care].* Zeist (external report).

Starbuck, E.D. (1899) *The Psychology of Religion. An Empirical Study of the Growth of Religious Consciousness.* New York: Charles Scribner's Sons.

Tepper, L., Rogers, S.A., Coleman, E.M. & Newton Malony, H. (2001) The Prevalence of Religious Coping among Persons with Persistent Mental Illness. *Psychiatric Services 52,* 660-665.

CHAPTER 1

MENTAL HEALTH AND RELIGION
A COMPLEX RELATIONSHIP

1. Mental health

In the last section of his principal work *Als ziende de Onzienlijke* ('As seeing Him who is invisible') (1974), the Dutch psychologist of culture and religion Han Fortmann has dealt elaborately with the relationship between religion and mental health. He begins by stating that mental health is not easily definable on a scientific level. In defining mental health, we have to realise its cultural relativity. What is strange and out of line in one culture may be an altogether normal way of behaviour in another. Therefore Fortmann points out that we must consider the function the behaviour has for the person, rather than the outward appearance. 'The hallucinations and the visions that Indians in California evoke in themselves through psychedelics and fasting, differ from the visions of psychotic patients in the function they have for the individual' (Fortmann 1974, 306). One and the same behaviour is an expression of a cultural habit in one case and an expression of a splintered personality in another. Moreover, in a certain culture ideological (political, philosophical and theological) presuppositions influence the concepts of what is mentally sane and what is not. Hence, many definitions of mental health have only relative or limited value. However, a number of definitions try to avoid these limitations by using a wide, open and/or relatively abstract formulation. In this manner Paloutzian (1983) defines mental health in terms of:
  – the absence of excessive feelings of guilt;
  – a realistic estimation and acceptance of one's shortcomings;
  – experiencing not too much or too little tension in one's life;
  – the ability to deal with problems;
  – leading a satisfactory social life;
  – having a sufficient amount of feelings of happiness.
Fortmann himself offers the following formulation:
  "The ability (freedom!) to realise oneself (e.g. in work) and to lose oneself... The term 'freedom' is not sufficient in itself. One should

add that it is a freedom that functions in two ways: self-actualisation and surrender" (Fortmann 1974, 361).

If we study the literature relating mental health to religion, it would seem that rather diverse subjects are brought together under the common denominator of mental health. Mental health can refer to (a) personal characteristics, (b) (deviant) social behaviour and (c) psychiatric or psychopathological issues. Personal characteristics can be traits such as dogmatism, authoritarianism, suggestibility and over-scrupulousness, from which we all suffer to some extent. Here the issue of mental health only arises if a person is excessively determined by such a characteristic. In the category of deviant social behaviour we find themes like alcoholism, drug addiction, criminality, sexual deviations, etc. In these cases the aspect of mental health is mainly related to the social stigma of these actions. In psychiatric or psychopathological cases (mental health in a stricter sense) the instability of the individual is highest. The milder neurotic disorders should be distinguished from the more serious psychotic ones that need professional (clinical) help in most cases. In the following section we will present some concrete examples of each category.

2. The complex interrelation between religion and mental health

Before addressing the relationship between religion and mental health, we want to state briefly how we will use the term 'religion' in this contribution. In defining religion, we make a distinction between substantial and functional definitions. Substantial definitions refer to a specific quality of religious phenomena. These substantial definitions usually derive their 'substance' from the Judeo-Christian tradition. At least there is a reference to a transcendent reality. Functional definitions concern the result that is brought about by religion. A frequently mentioned result is 'an answer to the ultimate questions of life'. This answer may be derived from God, or humanism, but it can also be found in interpersonal relationships, self-actualisation and enjoyment of life. We will not limit ourselves to a specific definition. However, since research in the psychology of religion is mainly situated in Judeo-Christian culture, references to a relationship with a transcendent, more or less personal God will be prevalent in the material to be dealt with.

In current literature simple relations between religion and mental health, such as Freud's (1927) statement that religion keeps man immature and consequently mentally unhealthy, can no longer be found. Most authors assume different possible relations between religion and mental health. Argyle & Beit-Hallahmi (1975) mention three possible relations. First, religion can enhance the individual's well-being and happiness. Second, religion can be seen as a form of psychopathology or at least as a factor leading to unadjusted behaviour in the individual. Third, emotionally unstable people can turn to religion in an attempt to rise above their problems.

Paloutzian (1983) lists four possible relations: 1. people with mental disorders become religious hoping to be able to control their problems; 2. religion makes originally healthy people unhealthy; 3. some forms of religion are pathogenic, other forms are beneficial to mental health; 4. there is no connection between religion and mental health.

According to Spilka *et al.* (1985) the relationship can be differentiated even further. Religion can:
1. cure the pathological by working as a *therapeuticum*;
2. repress the pathological by suppressing potential deviant behaviour through religious socialisation;
3. hide the pathological when religion becomes a haven to the individual;
4. express the pathological in a religious form;
5. cause the pathological when it is the cause of mental insanity.

As the latter categories differentiate the field of research best, we will now elaborate on it.

2.1. Religion as therapy

In the field of religion and belief, a large range of activities and experiences can be found that have an implicitly therapeutic function. Especially participation in *religious rituals* (confession, faith healing, exorcism, celebrations, pilgrimage etc.) can have considerable curative effects. Also *intense religious experiences* such as mystical experiences, speaking in tongues and conversion are well known for their therapeutic effects.

Although 'primitive' societies were more liable to have rituals than our modern industrialised society, some important rituals are still intact. One of the most important social functions of the church in our western society is to offer rituals concerning radical transitions in life such as birth, marriage, illness and death. Weekly church attendance may have decreased in frequency, but at occasions such as baptisms, weddings and funerals many citizens use the rituals the church has to offer. Since the church obviously meets a need in this respect, the question arises what function and effect these kinds of rituals have. Pieper (1988) has pointed out that the individual can benefit from a ritual in two ways. First, the ritual channels emotions, thus enhancing the individual's stability. It can allow for the expression of emotions that are not easily verbalised. To this end, the ritual uses well-known channels so that the individual is not overwhelmed by his or her emotions. In the case of a wedding this may be feelings of festivity and joy, in the case of a baptism feelings of wonder, in the case of a funeral feelings of meaninglessness and fear. In these cases, symbols within the ritual make it possible to come into contact with hidden fears and anxieties or with the archetypes (Jung) in the collective unconscious, in a non-threatening way.

Second, the ritual provides a frame of interpretation, thus guiding the concrete life situation by attributing a specific sense and meaning to it. In the case of a funeral this may be the Christian belief in an afterlife, implying a possible reunion with the deceased in the future. Rituals also facilitate the transition to a new role by providing a frame of explanation: an ideology legitimising the new role and explaining how to act within it. In discussing rites of initiation, Van der Hart (1984) points out that the tribe's myths and central symbols (the cosmology) are passed on to newcomers in these rites.

Elsewhere (Van der Hart 1981) he states that similar rituals may also be relevant outside of the religious domain, namely in the current practice of psychotherapy when initiating a transition to a new attitude to life. In close connection with this concept, Derks *et al.* (1991) have described pilgrimage as a transforming ritual. In addition to causing religious changes a pilgrimage can also have positive effects on a person's mental well-being. Research (Morris 1982; Van Uden & Pieper 1990; Pieper & Van Uden 1991) has shown the actual therapeutic effects of pilgrimages to Lourdes concerning the mental well-being of the pilgrims. Pilgrimages such as these evidently decrease feelings of anxiety and (partly also) depressive feelings. They also increase the relevance of the Christian meaning-giving system.

Let us now consider some intense religious experiences that may have a positive effect on the individual's psychosocial well-being, starting with the mystical experience. Boisen, who himself endured a number of psychotic episodes in his life, saw a close connection between certain forms of mental disorder and certain forms of mystical experience (Stroeken 1983). Boisen felt that such a mixture of psychotic/mystical experience is an attempt to overcome an imminent disintegration of the personality. In most cases the result is a constructive reorganisation, a restoration of the unity of the self. A quotation from an interview with a young woman conducted in another context offers insight in the depth of experiences such as these.

"I also think that in those days that I was doing very badly, that I spent in a padded cell, I was so scared that I was also a danger to myself, that I wanted to be dead... That I heard songs again just then... That was the only thing that gave me the feeling, that didn't abandon me, or something like that. Well, parts of psalms that came to mind suddenly. When things were really black, when I didn't know how to go on, then I always was told very joyfully: 'Count your blessings one by one'. Well, at a moment like this I didn't feel blessed at all, but they were very cheerful songs and darned, then all of a sudden I indeed had a blessing that I could count. And then 'Praise the Lord'. And that in itself was great of course, because that was quite something! Something to live for if only because it comes to your mind. Yes, yes, it was just enough to hold on to" (Pieper 1988, 74).

Here we have a religious/mystical experience that stops the disintegration of the personality. We borrow another example from the psychiatrist Gyselen's contribution to the volume *Hoe menselijk is mystiek?* ('How human is mysticism') (Gyselen *et al.* 1979). Gyselen described the life of a 52-year-old patient and the positive effect a mystical experience had in the course of the psychotherapeutic process.

"This turning point occurs during a walk on a road in the countryside. 'Suddenly a weight fell off me. I felt light. The air vibrated and had a heart that was beating. The trees were my allies. The bricks were living and trembling and were intensely colourful. One's heart beats on the rhythm of the vibrations all around, then. You feel one with all that is, and that all that is, is good. The colour of the clouds gave me a feeling of peace, nature knew me exactly... This occurrence, and I am inclined to say: this Divine occurrence, I would almost label it best as a Divine intervention in the earthly existence of the man who I was at that time. I can describe it best as a radical movement away from my 'I' as I had always experienced it, while the other

I was a spectator of my person. This new me felt absorbed, no, felt part of Something Who is cosmic, Who is now and always. Something real beyond description. I remember now that I saw myself and I was filled with disgust. And I also thought that in fact anyone who was interested could see me like this: full of sin, arrogance and vanity. And I understood that in my intellectual zeal to understand everything rationally, I in fact wanted to be my own God. And then it seemed as if I made a jump: a surrender to faith. The realisation that one doesn't necessarily have to understand everything with one's intellect but that one can live in peace and inner tranquillity, knowing with each and every fibre of one's body that since God is, everything is good. And that God supports the Life in me, me and everything and everything. And that I know another word synonymous to Life: Love – fiery. I think that this experience didn't last very long, maybe it was only a flash. But this nevertheless was enough to enjoy a kind of tranquillity for months that I had never known before. A tranquillity that started by seeing everything new…'" (Gyselen *et al.* 1979, 17-18).

Gyselen concluded that this experience could be interpreted as 'an attack on the illness' and that, from a psychological point of view, this mystical experience definitely did not make the patient more ill, but, quite to the contrary, had brought the patient closer to his true self.

Conversion is an experience in which there is a reintegration and transformation of the personality. People speak of a new self, a rebirth etc. A state of doubt and discomfort changes into a state of tranquillity and joy. Saint Augustine's story of his conversion is a perfect example of this experience. In the eighth book of his *Confessiones* he described his state of mind as follows:

"But as this deep meditation dredged all my wretchedness up from the secret profundity of my being and heaped it all together before the eyes of my heart, a huge storm blew up within me and brought on a heavy rain of tears." Augustine went to an isolated place and "Suddenly I heard a voice from a house nearby – perhaps a voice of some boy or girl, I do not know – singing over and over again, 'Pick it up and read, pick it up and read'". Augustine took the first passage from the Bible his eyes saw and he started to read (Rom. 13:13): "Not in dissipation and drunkenness, nor in debauchery and lewdness, nor in arguing and jealousy; but put on the Lord Jesus Christ, and make no provision for the flesh or the gratification of your desires" (Augustine 1998, 167-168).

The last subject we want to discuss is prayer. Clark (1958, 325) saw prayer as an 'inexpensive substitute for the psychiatrist's couch'. In the direct contact with God, one can ask for help, guidance and for-giveness of sins. In extreme crisis situations (such as war) even the most hardened atheist often resorts to prayer in one form or another. Irrespective of an actual intervention of God, from a psychological point of view, prayer can have a reassuring and liberating influence. Prayer then functions as a coping-mechanism: one tries to get a grip on a situation by attributing sense and meaning to it. Janssen, *et al.* (1989) have drawn similar conclusions from an empirical survey among 192 Dutch high school pupils:

"So, praying primarily seems to be a way of coping with inevitable, incurable unhappiness" (...) "Prayer can be seen as a way of constructing reality, as a way of making sense in a multi-interpretable world" (...) "We have defined praying as a verb, as an activity: praying is a mechanism to construct and interpret one's experience" (Janssen *et al.* 1989, 37).

2.2. Suppression of deviant behaviour by religious socialisation

Through a strict religious upbringing or socialisation, potentially devi-ant behaviour can be channelled into socially acceptable behaviour. It is well known for example that education in religious families often is aimed at controlling undesirable emotions such as anger and aggres-sion. This second function of religion will be most effective in coun-tries like the U.S. where socially acceptable standards coincide with religious standards. The suppression of deviant behaviour can be achieved in three ways.

First, the religious community can exercise a fundamental influ-ence on the individual by disapproving and punishing undesirable be-haviour and by encouraging and rewarding desirable behaviour. The closer the relationships between the members of the community, the more radically the individual can be 'shaped'. A well-known example of this influence is alcohol and drug abuse. In the U.S. many young people from traditional Protestant or Jewish families use much less alcohol and drugs than secularised youngsters of the same age group. We also find a strong group pressure within new religious movements (some based on Western, some based on Eastern religious and phi-losophical traditions). The press often points at the dangers connected to this. A review of psychological and psychiatric studies in this field (Richardson 1985) shows, however, that joining a community has a mainly beneficial effect on the health of the people that are concerned. Richardson has dealt with research regarding groups like the 'Jesus People', 'Ananda Marga', 'Unification Church' etc. His study showed that the social ties within the group effectively decreased neurotic phenomena and led to the resocialisation of young people who were alienated from social life before.

We find an example of this in Van der Lans' study *Volgelingen van de goeroe* ('Followers of the Guru') (1981). A 26-year-old man, who has been a member of the 'Divine Light Mission' for five years related as follows:

"I was totally obsessed with LSD and high all day long. I was into astrology, Gurdjieff, Uyldert, Hesse, Kerouac, Buddhism. I was searching terribly, I had no work, no study, very few friends." He had very little contact with his parents, even though they supported him financially. Because of the LSD he had got into an identity crisis: "My ego, all of my personality collapsed. It was as if I had to start all over again... I had clearly recognised the question in myself: What am I doing here? Why can't I function in this world like everybody else? I had really got a desire to get up in the morning and to go to work...". He then got in contact with the 'Divine Light Mission' through a friend. The 'premies', "with their short hair and their silly suits", to him were a weird company. "But then I got 'satsang'. Somebody was trying to communicate his experience. That was enough for me. I recognised it totally and felt that this was what I wanted." Since his initiation he had not used any drugs nor smoked cigarettes. The relationship with his parents was good now. "They think it's great that I look as neatly as this all of a sudden, with short hair. Apart from that they are not interested" (Van der Lans 1981, 56-57).

Second, not only the social pressure of the community of believers, but also the content of beliefs (dogmas and doctrines) can have a controlling effect. A good Christian has to live according to the Ten Commandments and many other doctrines of faith. With the addition of ideas of a punishing God, this can have a pervasive influence on social behaviour. Already in the nineteenth century the French sociologist Durkheim pointed to the relationship between religion and suicide. It has been hypothesised that Roman Catholic countries like Spain and Italy, where suicide is considered to be a mortal sin, would show considerably lower percentages of suicide than Protestant countries like

Great Britain and Iceland. It has to be mentioned however that Argyle & Beit-Hallahmi (1975) have compared the number of suicides in eighteen European countries in the year 1960 and have concluded that Durkheim's thesis did no longer hold.

The acquisition of desired behaviour can also occur through the imitation of religious models. Social learning theory states that imitation of models is one of the most important ways in which children acquire new styles of behaviour. Models may be found in the religious community (religious leaders, familiar pastors, ministers etc.) or in the religious tradition (biblical heroes, Jesus and his apostles, martyrs, saints etc.). In this context we also have to mention the social role theory of the Swedish psychologist of religion Sundén (1966). In describing religious experience, he referred to 'Rollen-übernahme' ('role taking') as a process in which one takes the roles of persons in biblical and other traditional religious stories.

2.3. Religion as a haven

A religious system can function as a haven, as a safe sanctuary that provides shelter against the tensions and troubles of daily life in a number of ways. Monastic life offers a regulated, controlled existence, providing protection against the vicissitudes of life outside the monastery's walls. Acceptance by a religious group can alleviate fears of social isolation and rejection. The belief in divine protection increases feelings of security. Let us look at a number of examples.

A study of Jehovah's Witnesses (Spencer 1975) showed that, compared to the general population, their rate of schizophrenia was three to four times higher. According to Spilka et al. (1985) Jehovah's Witnesses also tend to attract people looking for an ultra-traditional spiritual community with a strict moral code, thus hoping to find protection against the temptations of life.

In some cases members of new religious movements appear to have a past characterised by severe psychological problems, drug addiction, alcoholism, prostitution or criminality. Joining such a religious movement can be seen as an attempt to flee from that past. A quote from the aforementioned booklet Followers of the Guru (Van der Lans 1981) shows this clearly:

"What was the central point? How shall I put this? That I wanted to find God, that I wanted to be happy, that I wanted to know the meaning of my life; what is it all about? Actually everything was less important than this. I had disengaged myself from everything, my whole attention was fixated on this. I had abandoned my school, had left drama school, had gone from Amsterdam to South Limburg, because someone lived there who I felt could teach me something. I had given away all my possessions, my furniture, records, books. I had simply done away with it all. I had burnt my ships behind me" (Van der Lans 1981, 79).

Religious sects with strong, authoritarian leaders can also attract immature, dependent personalities. Galanter *et al.* (1979) concluded that about four in ten 'Moonies' (members of Rev. Moon's Unification Church) had serious psychological problems prior to joining this community. The search for a secure religious haven is not simple. Especially with sects and new religious movements we see a number of mentally unstable persons switching from one group to another. Their ties to a specific group are weak. The number of switches from one group to another seems to increase in accordance with the degree of mental insecurity of the people involved. It should be mentioned that most of the members of such groups function at a normal mental level. Often social circumstances, such as contacts with friends and acquaintances strongly influence the chances of participation in this kind of movements (Lofland & Stark 1965).

Monastic life too appears to have a considerable attraction for neurotic and prepsychotic people (Kurth 1961). Joining the group can however prevent admission to a mental hospital, but often the protective shield does not work for long. Kurth also found more cases of mental disturbance in enclosed orders (such as the Carmelites), than in the more socially active ones (orders involved in e.g. education like the Ursuline nuns). Judging by the following quote from the book *Nonnen* ('Nuns', Bernstein 1978), about a woman who entered a convent right after her mother's death, monastic life can also provide protection when coping with stressful life events:

"A woman who would have been rejected almost certainly with the tests of today entered the convent out of grief when her mother died, thirty years ago: 'I was eighteen and very sad and upset. And as soon as the doors closed behind me I felt at ease, I knew I was in the right place'" (Bernstein 1978, 70).

2.4. Religion as an expression of mental disorder

Religion can enable the individual to express mental aberration as it were in a 'masked' way. Eccentric behaviour can be permitted within the context of a religious system. The individual will probably be regarded as different and peculiar, but the label 'mentally disturbed' will not be attached to him or her openly.

Some descriptions of mystical experiences are very similar to descriptions of the behaviour of patients with severe mental disturbances. An example, taken from Antoon Vergote's study *Bekentenis en begeerte in de religie* ('Guilt and desire in religion') (1978) can clarify this:

"The Venerable Agnes Blannbekin, born in Vienna towards the end of the thirteenth century, was totally obsessed with the question of what actually happened to the 'Holy Foreskin' of Jesus, an issue that was discussed by some theologians in those days, in the context of the question whether the resurrected body would be violated or not. God ended Agnes' agonising worries by revealing to her that our Lord brought the foreskin back to life with him on the day of his resurrection. Fortunately God did not add that he was about to reveal to Saint Birgitta that the holy foreskin was still hidden in... Rome. For Agnes this revelation was the start of a sequence of remarkable ecstasies, which were reported by her 'unworthy father confessor', as the Franciscan Ermenic introduced himself. So we see how Agnes in one year, when on the day of the circumcision she was crying bitterly as usual, started to contemplate where the foreskin of the Lord could be, even though she had already been told this in the revelation. Now hark. 'Soon she felt a tiny skin on her tongue, like the skin of an egg but softer, and this tiny little skin she swallowed. When she had swallowed it, she felt this extremely tiny skin on her tongue again, just like before, and so she swallowed it once more. And this occurred to her a hundred times indeed... The sweetness accompanying the digestion was so strong that she sensed a delightful transformation in all her limbs and joints. During this revelation she was filled with an inner light in such a way, that she could observe herself totally'. The Lord favoured her still more with innumerable tender and chaste touches of his hand or with a lamb coming from the altar. Every time God visited her 'Agnes was filled with an excitement in her chest that was so intense that it went through her body and that it burnt as a result, not in a painful but in a most pleasurable manner'. No wonder the blood letter one time was astonished when he let her blood, because the girl's blood was so hot that it was boiling" (Vergote 1978, 261-262).

This is an illustration of the fact that a religious experience can raise suspicions of mental insanity. For that matter, well-known mystics like St. Teresa have also sometimes been depicted as hysterics. Jeanne d'Arc has been diagnosed as a paranoid and schizophrenic, among other things, and Dostoyevsky and the apostle Paul have sometimes been classified as epileptics.

Glossolalia (speaking in tongues) too can in some cases refer to an underlying pathology. During meetings of the Pentecostal movement, speaking in tongues functions as an emotional confession. The sounds that are produced by the 'tongue-speakers' are usually meaningless. It consists of strings of vowels and consonants that are expressed in an emotional tone of voice coupled with rhythmic movements of the body. These sounds cannot be identified as any known language, apart from fragments from the Bible that are often mixed into it. Goodman (1972) argued that the normal cortical control of language production stops, because of the extreme emotional excitement (e.g. when during mass meetings a charismatic religious leader urges the participants to set themselves free), and that lower subcortical centres of the brain take over the production of language. In this case unconscious personal problems can also be at work. Vroon (1978) related speaking in tongues to the Tourette syndrome, which is characterised by an uncontrolled and distorted expression of cursing and coarseness.

In 1 Corinthians 14:5-14, Paul warns against the phenomenon of speaking in tongues: "Now, I wish for you all to speak in tongues, but even more for you to prophesy. The one who prophesies is greater than the one who speaks in tongues unless he interprets it so that the community may be built up. Now, brothers, if I came to you speaking in tongues, how would I benefit you unless I also spoke to you with revelation or knowledge, with prophecy or with teachings? ...So if you do not produce intelligible speech by the tongue, how then will one understand what is being said? You will then be speaking to the wind... if I do not understand the meaning of the language, I am a barbarian to the one who is speaking to me and he to me. So you also, since you are zealous for ecstasy of the spirit, must strive diligently for the up building of the community through this as much as possible. Therefore, let the one who speaks in tongues pray that he may also interpret. For if I pray in tongues, my spirit may be praying, but my mind is good for nothing." Paul here points to the dangers of what he calls "the enchantment of the spirit". An interpretation, a translation is necessary.

Scrupulosity is the third phenomenon that can clarify how the pathological can be expressed in the religious. We speak of scrupulosity when an individual experiences continuous doubt and insecurity about sin and guilt and is absorbed by the question whether he is breaking some rule. This obsession triggers compulsive and ritualised actions that are meant to control doubt and insecurity. The religious ritual can fill the need for such compulsive actions. Until recently, especially in the Roman Catholic Church believers were supposed to strictly observe ritual rules. For example, many conditions had to be fulfilled before one could receive Holy Communion. As early as 1907 Freud pointed to the relationship between individual compulsive actions and collective religious rituals. He mentioned the following similarities between compulsive actions and religious ritual: 1. the moral dilemma that arises when the actions are neglected; 2. the conscientious way in which they are performed; 3. the fact that these actions are isolated from other daily activities; 4. the fact that interruptions are forbidden. Freud ended his argument with the following conclusion that antagonised generations of theologians and believers. "According to these similarities and analogies it could be ventured to understand obsessive compulsive neurosis as the pathological counterpart of religious development, to define neurosis as an individual religiosity; to define religion as a universal obsessive compulsive neurosis" (Freud 1907, 21). Religion is a collective obsessive compulsive neurosis, which can save on an individual neurosis; again we see how the psychological problem (the neurosis) is expressed through the religious domain.

The final possible expression of mental disturbance through religion we mention here concerns the priesthood. Personality disorders can sometimes make people think that they are destined for the priesthood. Mental troubles can motivate people to turn to clerical life as an outlet for emotional problems. This may be the case for instance when celibacy becomes a cover-up for problems with sexuality and intimacy. Some authors report that the number of mental disturbances among the clergy is higher than among the average population. Kennedy et al. (1977) identified 65% of a sample of Roman Catholic priests as being sociopsychologically either maldeveloped or underdeveloped. The question is of course what is cause and what is effect. Research by Hoenkamp-Bisschops (1991) shows how compulsory celibacy can lead to all kinds of problematic behaviour. Nowadays it seems that only few people can cope with a celibate life style in a healthy way.

2.5. Religion as a hazard to mental health

Finally it is also possible that religion and faith in God present a hazard to mental health, causing mental dysfunctioning or increasing mental problems. The latter is the case when the function of a haven and that of expression go together with a loss of sense of reality to such a degree that possible non-religious therapeutic interventions are refused. God is then played off against the therapist who, because of his inferior status, can only be second best compared to an omniscient and omnipotent entity. Religious tradition provides many possibilities, like miracles, prophetic predictions, original sin, punishment by God like the destruction of Sodom and Gomorra, which patients embrace gladly to legitimise or continue their mental disorder or deviant behaviour. In his study *The three Christs of Ypsilanti* Rokeach (1964) described the confrontation between three psychiatric patients who are all convinced to be the true incarnation of Christ. For two years they were exposed to each other's convictions. At the end all three were still convinced to be Christ, thus revealing their rigid thinking and inability to change positively. Generally speaking, even in cases of not strictly pathological problems, there is the danger that religion may prevent the necessary confrontation with reality, if it is functioning as the 'opium of the people'. As a temporary sedation it is not so bad, but as a permanent anaesthesia it will cause destructive stagnation. However, the following case shows that there is only a thin line between sedation and stagnation. A widower, Mr Cox was interviewed in the context of a research project regarding the function of faith in the process of mourning:

"In his current religiosity his deceased wife has taken up an important place: 'The devotion of Our Lady comes back to me, but my wife, she stands above her. Because she is next to God, I wouldn't dare to use God's name in the second place, so my wife comes second and my heavenly mother Mary third, let me say it this way, and I beg her every day to help me'. According to Mr Cox contact with the Supreme Being is possible, but only through a mediator: 'For me, that is my wife, she is my mediator. I still have contact with her often, so I let it all run through her. And then I get information, I have it right here on paper, about 380 pages already. I keep a regular record of it, the things that she predicts to me or that she dictates. Because I am in spiritual contact with her, this is possible. I used to be able to summon her myself. Then I went to her grave and spoke with her. Then I heard her voice and she gave me advice.' Every year Mr Cox commemorates the passing away of his wife: 'These weeks, well, they are horrible moments for me. I experience everything again. This year I ran out of the house. My table in the living room was covered with candles and flowers and her picture was in the middle. The candles burned there all day.' In this 'remembrance week' he does not want to be disturbed. In a wall unit Mr Cox has installed a kind of home altar: 'It has a niche, and in it are six candles and her large picture. On my desk I have a picture, on my drawer too. For as long as I shall live, I've promised her, I will put flowers with them. Up to today I have done so. On my desk a small candle is burning all day long. I'd rather not talk about it very much, because I will never forget it'" (Van Uden 1985, 53-54). Here the adoration of his wife as a saint, a neurotic form of fear regulation, helps Mr Cox to survive, but only at the expense of a considerable amount of his freedom.

Religion can also cause mental problems by itself. Freud argued that in the battle between Id and Superego religion takes the side of the Superego. Religious commandments and prohibitions are intended to restrain sexual and aggressive impulses. Since religion is aiming at moral perfection, trespassing these laws will cause feelings of guilt and sin. In extreme cases this can lead to compulsive guilt feelings that can dominate and paralyse an individual's life. Furthermore, this can lead to often extreme penitence varying from the thrashing out of sin by flagellants in the Middle Ages to public confessions of guilt in our current TV era.

In the Netherlands Aleid Schilder (1987) has researched the issue of guilt and sin. Her study *Hulpeloos maar schuldig* ('Helpless yet guilty'), regarding the members of a strict orthodox Dutch-Reformed Church, provided some insight in the paralysing effect guilt feelings can have on people's thinking and doing. She showed how doctrines like 'you are burdened with original sin, and you can do nothing against it' can cause or intensify depression as an expression of "learned helplessness" (Seligman). A passage from a diary of a client looking back at her depression shows how these factors are interrelated:

"In our church sin is constantly preached about, that you can't do anything by yourself, that you are a miserable human being, that you can't do anything good out of yourself. And that was emphasised so much, and at home (i.e. in the past A.S.) ditto. When you have heard that you are a miserable person, you become programmed like that. I think that God's love and mercy are not enough talked about; feelings are never allowed. But I do have feelings, a whole lot. As I had to learn with my mind that I was a miserable person, my feeling could do nothing else but feel miserable!" (Schilder 1987, 76-77).

On a cognitive level religion can also be a hazard to mental health. The emphasis on obedience and blind faith may enhance immaturity and unrealistic thinking. When religion provides simple, uncomplicated solutions for complicated problems of life, it encourages unrealistic attitudes. Both aspects (obedience and the intolerance of ambiguity) are found in so-called authoritarian personalities. These authoritarian personalities can cause considerable damage to society when they are organised in groups like the Ku Klux Klan. In extreme cases such an absolute obedience can lead to calamities like the mass suicide in Jonestown (Guyana) in 1978. Jim Jones led 912 members of his sect (the People's Temple Movement) into death. We borrow a dramatic description of this event from Conway & Siegelman (1979).

"Then Jones addressed the people of Jonestown and told them that the member of congress and the journalists were dead and that the military forces of Guyana were on their way to Jonestown to torture and kill the inhabitants of the commune. 'It is time to die in dignity', Jones said, thus for the last time repeating a vow that he had taken often before: to lead his followers into a 'mass suicide for the glory of socialism'. Then, on Jones' orders, the temple doctor and his medical team brought to the front a battered washing tub filled with strawberry lemonade that had been mixed with large quantities of cyanide, tranquillisers and analgesics. Jones told the gathering: 'The time has come to meet each other in a new place. Bring the babies first', he ordered; and his nurses injected the poison into their throats. Then the rest of them came to the front, complete families at once, every one drank a cup of poison and was guided away by the temple guards and forced to lie down in rows, facing down. Within a few minutes the people started to gasp for air, as blood was flowing out of their mouth and nose, until the last convulsive movements started. According to witnesses the ritual lasted for almost five hours. All through this time Jim Jones was seated on his high chair in the pavilion and repeated: 'I have tried, I have tried, I have tried'. And then: 'Mother, Mother, Mother, Mother'. When it was all over, Jones was lying on the platform face forward, with a bullet through his head. And 912 people were dead" (Conway & Siegelman 1979, 245).

3. Explaining the differences in effect

The five possible connections between religion and mental health that we have dealt with in the second section can be divided into two global parts. In the first four cases religion has a positive effect: healing, suppressing pathology, softening pathology by providing a haven and by expressing pathology. It is questionable, however, whether this softening is beneficial in the end. In the fifth case the relation is a negative one. This division into two categories is quite common in the empirical research that has been performed over the last decades. Based on a meta-analysis of 24 studies on psychopathology, Bergin (1983) concludes that religion can sometimes be related to psychopathology and sometimes to mental health.

In order to explain the differences in the results of the various studies we have to discuss a number of methodological questions. First, most empirical studies are interested in the correlation between religion and mental health. This type of research can establish a connection, a correlation, but it cannot establish the direction of the connection: if we assume that the relationship is negative, it cannot be established what is the cause and what is the effect (the old question: what came first, the chicken or the egg?). If we assume that pathology came first, religion can be seen as the expression of pathology. If, however, we assume that religion came first, then religion can be seen as the cause of the disturbances.

Second, it is very difficult to compare the various studies, because the ways in which 'religion' and 'mental health' are defined and measured differ. Concerning religion, questions can be asked about religious beliefs (which have a range of varieties), but also about religious experiences or about religious behaviours like church attendance. In order to measure mental health, huge handbooks full of tests and instruments can be consulted focusing on aspects of mental health such as anxiety, depression, self-esteem, authoritarianism, self-ideal/self-discrepancy etc.

Third, intervening variables can have a confusing influence. This is the case when an established relation between religion and mental health is actually caused by a third variable (the intervening one), which is related to both religion and mental health, forging them together. An example of such a variable is socio-economic class: when people from a low socio-economic class can be characterised by having both an authoritarian style of childrearing and by being very religious, chances are that the children from this class will be both very authoritarian and very religious. Research regarding children in this class may lead to the wrong conclusion that highly religious people are authoritarian. This conclusion is wrong because the established relation has actually been caused by the fact that an authoritarian style of upbringing and religiosity go together in this class. Other variables of this kind are gender, education, age and ethnic origin. Research projects, therefore, will have to deal with the possible influence of such intervening variables and will have to control for their effects in the analysis of data.

Apart from these answers, which refer to influences of the methodology used, another answer can be given to explain the differences in the various studies concerning the relation between religion and mental health. Even if all methodological obstacles could be avoided, the relation would still be twofold, as essentially there are two forms of religion: healthy and unhealthy religion. The former is related to healthy, the latter to unhealthy personal and social characteristics. There is a parallel here with the well-known distinction between intrinsic and extrinsic religion. In the intrinsic form, religion is valuable in itself and goes together with personal adjustment. In the extrinsic form, religion is a means for other purposes, such as security and social status and it goes together with a non-balanced personality. Baker & Gorsuch (1982) actually have established differences between intrinsic and extrinsic believers: the former scored lower on a number of anxiety indicators such as ego weakness and paranoid feelings. Spilka et al. (1985, 315) draw the following conclusion in this respect:

"A faith that provides an open-minded, competent guide for everyday living is found in conjunction with good adjustment and effective coping behavior. A shallow, externalised religion that is needed when things aren't what one desires is more likely to be a correlate of shortcomings in personality and social interaction."

Again the question comes to mind as to what is the cause and what is the effect. Does a mentally healthy person develop an intrinsic religiosity or does intrinsic religion cause mental health? It is possible that the relation is twofold, in other words that the variables of religion and person can be both effect and cause. An example centred on images of God may illustrate the former. It appears that disordered people develop 'disordered' images of God. The God in question is either threatening or punishing or avenging, or the image of God is unclear and confused. Both these images of God have negative effects on mental health. In the first case feelings of guilt and sin increase, causing the feeling of self-esteem to sink even deeper. In the second case life is deprived of sense and meaning. This downward spiral can be stopped, however, by profound and radical religious experiences, such as mystical experiences or conversion, but also by experiences around birth, love, illness and death. Then, instead of the negative image of God, a loving and forgiving God appears, causing a positive effect on mental health through an increased feeling of self-confidence and self-esteem.

To summarise, the relation between religion and mental health is a complex one. This complexity is related to the fact that individuals can deal in a different way with forms of religion that are provided by the culture. Whether, from a psychological point of view, religion is healing or not, will depend on its functioning in the individual's total mental economy (Van Uden 1985). As James (1994/1902) put it: ultimately healthy religion can only be recognised by the fruits it yields.

References

Argyle, M. & Beit-Hallahmi, B. (1975) *The Social Psychology of Religion.* London: Routledge and Kegan Paul.

Augustine (1998) *The Confessions* (Transl. Maria Boulding OSB). New York: Vintage Books (Vintage Spiritual Classics).

Baker, M. & Gorsuch, R. (1982). Trait Anxiety and Intrinsic-Extrinsic Religiousness. *Journal for the Scientific Study of Religion 21*, 119-122.

Bergin, A.E. (1983) Religiosity and Mental Health. A Critical Reevaluation and Meta-Analysis. *Professional Psychology: Research and Practice 14*, 170-184.

Bernstein, M. (1978) *Nonnen. Van een mysterieus bestaan achter kloostermuren naar de emancipatie van een oude levensstijl. [Nuns. From a Mysterious Existence behind Convent Walls to the Emancipation of an Old Life Style].* Baarn: In den Toren.

Boisen, A.T. (1952) The General Significance of Mystical Identification in Cases of Mental Disorder. *Psychiatry 15*, 287-296.

Clark, W.H. (1958) *The Psychology of Religion.* New York: Macmillan.

Conway, F. & Siegelman, J. (1979) *Knappen [Snapping]*. Amsterdam/Brussel: Elsevier.

Derks, F., Pieper, J. & Uden, van M. (1991). Transformatie en confirmatie. Interviews met bedevaartgangers naar Wittem en Lourdes [Transformation and Confirmation. Interviews with Pilgrims to Wittem and Lourdes]. In: Uden, van M., Pieper, J. & Henau, E. (eds.) *Bij Geloof. Over bedevaarten en andere uitingen van volksreligiositeit [Faith or Superstition? On Pilgrimages and Other Forms of Popular Religion]*. Hilversum: Gooi en Sticht, 105-123.

Fortmann, H.M.M. (1974) *Als ziende de Onzienlijke (deel 1 en 2) [As Seeing Him Who is Invisible (Vols. 1 and 2)]*. Hilversum: Gooi en Sticht.

Freud, S. (1907) *Zwangshandlungen und Religionsübungen [Obsessive Actions and Religious Practices]*. Freud Studienausgabe, 1975, Band 7, 11-21. Frankfurt: Fischer Verlag.

Freud, S. (1927) *Die Zukunft einer Illusion [The Future of an Illusion]*. Gesammelte Werke, 1961, Band 14, London.

Galanter, M., Rabkin, R., Rabkin, J. & Deutsch, A. (1979) The Moonies. A Psychological Study of Conversion and Membership in a Contemporary Religious Sect. *American Journal of Psychiatry 136*, 165-169.

Goodman, F.D. (1972) *Speaking in Tongues. A Cross-Cultural Study of Glossolalia*. Chicago: University of Chicago Press.

Gyselen, M. (1979). Mijn patiënt was meer dan ziek [My Patient was More than Just Ill]. In: Gyselen, M. *et al. Hoe menselijk is mystiek? [How Human is Mysticism?]*. Baarn: Ambo.

Hart, van der O. *et al.* (1981) *Afscheidsrituelen in psychotherapie [Leavetaking Rituals in Psychotherapy]*. Baarn: Ambo.

Hart, van der O. (1984) *Rituelen in psychotherapie. Overgang en bestendiging. [Rituals in Psychotherapy. Transition and Confirmation]*. Deventer: Van Loghum Slaterus.

Hoenkamp, A. (1991) *Varianten van celibaatsbeleving. Een verkennend onderzoek rond ambtscelibaat en geestelijke gezondheid. [Varieties of Celibacy Experience. An Exploratory Investigation of Official Celibacy and Mental Health]*. Baarn: Ambo.

James, W. (1902) *The Varieties of Religious Experience. A Study in Human Nature*. New York: Modern Library Press, 1994 (original 1902).

Janssen, J., Hart, de J. & Draak, den C. (1989) Praying Practices. *Journal of Empirical Theology 2*, 28-39.

Kennedy, E.C. *et al.* (1977). Clinical Assessment of a Profession. Roman Catholic Clergyman. *Journal of Clinical Psychology 33*, 120-128.

Kurth, C.J. (1961) Psychiatric and Psychological Selection of Candidates for the Sisterhood. *Guild of Catholic Psychiatrists Bulletin 8*, 19-25.

Lans, van der J. (1981) *Volgelingen van de goeroe. Hedendaagse religieuze bewegingen in Nederland [Followers of the Guru. Present-Day Religious Movements in the Netherlands]*. Baarn: Ambo.

Lofland, J. & Stark, R. (1965) Becoming a World Saver. A Theory of Conversion to a Deviant Perspective. *American Sociological Review 30*, 862-874.

Morris, P.A. (1982) The Effect of Pilgrimage on Anxiety, Depression and Religious Attitude. *Psychological Medicine 12*, 291-294.

Paloutzian, R.F. (1983) *Invitation to the Psychology of Religion.* Glenview: Scott/Foresman.

Pieper, J.Z.T. (1988) *God gezocht en gevonden? Een godsdienstpsychologisch onderzoek rond het kerkelijk huwelijk met pastoraaltheologische consequenties [God Searched and Found? Research in the Psychology of Religion regarding Church Weddings, with Pastoral Theological Consequences].* Nijmegen: Dekker & van de Vegt.

Pieper, J. & Uden, van M. (1991) De huidige Lourdesbedevaart. Motieven en effecten [Present-Day Pilgrimage to Lourdes. Motives and Effects]. In: Uden, van M. & Pieper, J. (eds.) *Bedevaart als volksreligieus ritueel. [Pilgrimage as a Popular Religious Ritual].* Heerlen: UTP-teksten 16, 7-26.

Richardson, J.T. (1985) Psychological and Psychiatric Studies of New Religions. In: Brown, L.B. *Advances in the Psychology of Religion.* Oxford: Pergamon, 209-223.

Rokeach, M. (1964) *The Three Christs of Ypsilanti.* New York: Knopf.

Schilder, A. (1987) *Hulpeloos maar schuldig. Het verband tussen een gereformeerde paradox en depressie [Helpless Yet Guilty. The Relation between a Reformed Paradox and Depression].* Kampen: Kok.

Spencer, J. (1975) The Mental Health of Jehovah's Witnesses. *British Journal of Psychiatry 126*, 556-559.

Spilka, B., Hood, R.W. & Gorsuch, R.L. (1985) *The Psychology of Religion. An Empirical Approach.* Englewood Cliffs, NY: Prentice Hall.

Stroeken, H. (1983) *Psychoanalyse, godsdienst en Boisen [Psychoanalysis, Religion and Boisen].* Kampen: Kok.

Sundén, H. (1966) *Die Religion und die Rollen. Eine psychologische Untersuchung der Frömmigkeit [Religion and Roles. A Psychological Investigation of Piety].* Berlin: Töpelmann.

Uden, van M.H.F. (1985) *Religie in de crisis van de rouw. Een exploratief onderzoek d.m.v. diepte-interviews [Religion in the Crisis of Mourning. An Exploratory Investigation through Depth Interviews].* Nijmegen: Dekker & van de Vegt.

Uden, van M. (1988) *Rouw, religie en ritueel [Mourning, Religion and Ritual].* Baarn: Ambo.

Uden, van M.H.F. & Pieper, J.Z.T. (1990) Christian Pilgrimage. Motivational Structures and Ritual Functions. In: Heimbrock, H.G. & Boudewijnse, H.B. (eds.) *Current Studies on Rituals. Perspectives for the Psychology of Religion.* Amsterdam/Atlanta: Rodopi, 165-176.

Vergote, A. (1978) *Bekentenis en begeerte in de religie. Psychoanalytische verkenning*. Antwerpen: De Nederlandsche Boekhandel. [Vergote, A. (1987) *Guilt and Desire. Religious Attitudes and their Pathological Derivations* [Transl. M.H. Wood], New Haven/London: Yale University Press.]

Vroon, P. (1978) *Stemmen van vroeger. Ontstaan en ontwikkeling van het zelfbewustzijn [Voices of Yore. Origins and Development of Self-Consciousness]*. Baarn: Ambo.

CHAPTER 2

RELIGION IN MENTAL HEALTH CARE: PATIENTS' VIEWS

1. Introduction

In the study reported below, the concepts 'worldview' and 'religion' have been defined as follows. 'Worldview' refers to the whole of values, standards and ideas people use when thinking of the meaning and purpose of life. We speak of 'religion' when these values, standards and ideas, as a whole or in part, derive from an existing religious institution (for instance Roman Catholicism or Protestantism). For most people who have participated in our study, their worldview is a religious one.

In the last years in the Netherlands the interest for the relation between worldview and religion on the one hand and social and mental health care on the other hand is growing. Firstly, we can point at a series of publications about this topic (Bauduin 1991; Den Draak & Kleingeld 1991; Kerssemakers 1989; Molenkamp 1994; Schilder & Schippers 1990; Vellenga 1992). Secondly, there are a growing number of conferences featuring this relation (Filius & Visch 1991; Visch 1991). Thirdly, a number of documents about policies and strategies for managing these issues in mental health care institutions have been published (Easton 1990; Riagg en Religie 1991).

In the discussion (and from now on we will focus on the regional community mental health care institutions in the Netherlands, called Riagg) two central premises are found. In the first place one agrees that religion and worldview could and should have a prominent place in many psychotherapeutic interventions. The physical, emotional, behavioural and social problems that the client brings in, are often related to their systems of meaning and their religious attitudes. In the second place, at the same time psychotherapists are being accused of neglecting this dimension. Some authors, in particular those who are close to the humanistic tradition, are especially concerned about neglecting worldview in general (Dijkhuis & Mooren 1988). Others, in particular those who are close to the Protestant tradition, are especially concerned about neglecting the religious values of clients (Schilder 1991a; 1991b; Van der Wal 1991). In the latter group are also authors who argue that pastoral workers should be working in the institutions for regional community mental health care, and even authors who advocate founding new regional community mental health care institutions, based on Christian principles. Some years ago they have had some success, because the Dutch government was financially supporting such an institution based on Christian principles (called the Gliagg).

2. Empirical research

Is there any empirical evidence, with respect to the institutions of regional community mental health care in the Netherlands, which supports these premises? We only know of Den Draak's (1990) limited pilot study, based on four interviews with psychotherapists, working in community mental health care agencies, and of De Groen & Slockers-Beverwijk's (1987) doctoral thesis. There is also a global inventory by the community mental health care agencies themselves (Nvagg 1989). This inventory was aiming only at institutions in Protestant regions. The main questions were: to what extent do your clients ask for treatment regarding religious and existential aspects of their problems, and is there enough expertise within the institution regarding the religious backgrounds of the clients?

Because of the lack of empirical evidence, we started in 1989 a research project among Riagg psychotherapists. The main conclusion of this inquiry – and this is consistent with the results of the Nvagg research – is that psychotherapists do pay attention to religious and worldview aspects of mental problems. There seems to be no massive aversion to discussing religious and worldview problems in treatment (Van der Lans et al. 1993). But these are the opinions of the psychotherapists. How do the clients themselves evaluate their treatment? In order to get an answer, we questioned in 1992 about 425 former clients of the Heerlen Riagg (situated in a mainly Roman Catholic region) and about 330 former clients of the Zwolle Riagg (situated in a highly Protestant region) (Pieper & Van Uden 1993a; 1993b). The questions were directed at three main areas. In the first place we asked about the ways in which religion and worldview are related to mental problems: is there any relation, and if so, is this a positive or negative one? Secondly, we asked about the ways in which therapists had reacted to these religious and worldview dimensions: had they been dealt with as relevant to the therapy or had they been avoided? Thirdly, we asked some questions about the wishes and needs of the former clients regarding the roles religious and worldview dimensions should play during therapy.

3. Results

3.1. Relations between religion/worldview and mental problems

Eight questions were used to measure the relation between religion/worldview and mental problems. One of the questions indicates a neutral relation, five of them indicate a negative relation and two a positive one. The following table shows the percentages of former clients who fully or partially agree with each question. The first figure represents the answers of the former clients of the Zwolle Riagg, the second one the opinions of the former clients of the Heerlen Riagg.

Table 1: *Relations between religion/worldview and mental problems*

		Zwolle/Heerlen*
1	My religion/worldview has influenced my problems.	43 / 43
2	My problems have been intensified because of my religion/worldview.	34 / 36
3	My religion/worldview has caused my problems.	15 / 27
4	My problems were related to my losing the religion/worldview of my childhood.	18 / 24
5	My religion/worldview has had a negative influence because of the emphasis put on values like humility, servitude and sacrifice.	23 / 30
6	My religion/worldview has had a negative influence because of the emphasis put on guilt and feelings of guilt.	28 / 31
7	Without my religion/worldview my problems would have been worse.	24 / 23
8	My religion/worldview has been a great support to me in dealing with my problems.	39 / 39

* percentages of clients who fully or partially agree

In general it can be stated that a considerable minority replied that their religion/worldview was in one way or another related to their mental problems. A factor analysis showed that a distinction could be made with reference to the relation experienced between religion/worldview and the problems of the respondents. Two factors have been found. The first factor contained those items referring to the negative influence of religion/worldview (intensify, cause, loss of religion, humility, guilt). In this factor the neutral item was to be found also ('religion/worldview has influenced my problems'). The second factor contained those items referring to the positive influence of religion/worldview (support, 'without it my problems would have been worse').

First, we will consider the negative influence in more detail. Some authors emphasise that excesses in religious education cause or continue mental problems. The book 'Helpless yet guilty' (Schilder 1987) gives an example with respect to the situation in the Netherlands. The author argues in the context of a Calvinist denomination, that feelings of guilt can indeed paralyse people, and that the message 'you are burdened with sin, and you can't do anything about it' can cause or strengthen a depression as a result of a "learned helplessness" process (according to Seligman's theory). We also have to point out the impact of evoking feelings of fear in religious education. Conformation to the severe (especially sexual) standards of the church was enforced by the fear of Doomsday, Hell and damnation and expulsion from the community. These feelings of fear can turn into phobias or deepen already existing phobic tendencies. Especially regarding women we can point at the emphasis that has been put (and sometimes still is being put) on humility, servitude and sacrifice, for which the Virgin Mary is the prime example.

What does the research show? In the questionnaire various degrees of negative influence on mental problems have been presented. 43% of the respondents agreed with the item 'my religion/worldview has influenced my problems'. For the item 'My problems have been intensified because of my religion/worldview' the agreement had receded to 34% (36%) and for the item 'my religion/worldview has caused my problems' to 15% (27%). With respect to the latter it has to be mentioned that the respondents mostly chose the alternative 'partially agree'. Nevertheless, more than one-seventh (Zwolle) or a quarter (Heerlen) of the respondents agreed that the cause of their problems was at least to some extent related to religion/worldview.

Two more detailed questions asked about the negative influence of religion in relation to the emphasis put, in past religious education, on humility, servitude and sacrifice on the one hand, and on guilt and feelings of guilt on the other hand. Regarding 'humility', 23% (30%) agreed that it had had (at least a partial) negative influence. Regarding guilt, this was 28% (31%). For example, a client made the following comment: "I think I had too strong principles. I could forgive neither my own mistakes nor the mistakes of other people. I was raised by my grandmother with ideas of Hell and Satan. In my childhood I developed a strong sense of guilt and a lot of fears, and I still have a strong awareness of sin."

It is often said that religion/worldview influences mental problems in particular in women, more specifically in a negative way, because of the emphasis in women's religious education on 'humility, servitude and sacrifice' and on 'guilt and feelings of guilt'. For that reason we investigated the possibility of a relation between the questions asked and gender. In Zwolle we found no relation. In Heerlen significantly more women than men replied that religion had had a negative influence in relation to the emphasis on 'humility, servitude and sacrifice' and on 'guilt and feelings of guilt'.

It is also possible that religious education leads to a religion/worldview that can function as a healing power. Without religion/worldview, the mental problems would have been more serious. Trust in a loving and forgiving God, trust in a God who helps people can give courage and strength to cope with imminent mental problems or limit the already existent problems. The parish community can offer security and social support that enable the individual to endure hardship. In this respect two questions were asked. For 39% (39%) of the respondents religion/worldview had been a great support in dealing with the problems; 24% (23%) replied that the problems would have been more serious without religion/worldview. This can be illustrated by a remark from a client: "I have got a lot of strength from Scripture texts like 1 Timothy 6:19. I very much like Psalm 38, the prayer of someone repentant. It is very up to date, a real beauty. Especially the Book of Proverbs offers a lot of practical help to all kinds of people, however different their backgrounds may be."

It has to be noted that the effect of religion being the cause of the problems doesn't exclude the possibility of religion being a huge support to people. This was the case for 16 (35) respondents out of 38 (78) who agreed that religion (partially) has been the cause of their problems. For these respondents religion had been the cause of their mental problems, while at the same time their religion had had healing effects on these problems.

Are there any differences between groups of respondents as regards the influence of religion/worldview? First, it appears that religious education was connected with the actual influence (positive as well as negative) of religion/worldview on mental problems. The stronger the religious education, the stronger it was connected with mental problems. Secondly, if religion and worldview influenced the mental problems of the clients, then this implies an important role of religion and worldview in the other parts of the respondents' lives. The belief that God pays personal attention was especially related to the experience that religion/worldview was a great support in dealing with problems. This also applied to church attendance. The more frequently one attended church, the more one found support. Thirdly, there was a correlation between experiencing support and the variable 'religious affiliation' (see Table 2). Because of the homogeneity of the Roman Catholic population in Heerlen, we will focus on the data from the research in Zwolle.

Table 2: *Relation between religious affiliation and experience of religious support*

	without religion my problems would have been worse	*religion has been a (great) support*
	% (partially) agree	*% (partially) agree*
Roman Catholic	22	38
Dutch Reformed	24	40
Calvinist	44	62
other denominations	55	73
no religion	6	15
average	24	39

(Chi^2= 32.07; sign.: 0.000; n= 249) (Chi^2= 36.69; sign.: 0.000; n= 250)

Especially the more orthodox (one should bear in mind that by 'other denominations' we refer to the more orthodox Protestant groups) and Calvinist religious groups found support and comfort in God. Finally age was connected with the following two variables: 'humility, servitude and sacrifice' and 'without religion the problems would have been worse'. Especially the elderly gave as their view that they had suffered from the emphasis put on humility, servitude and sacrifice

and (at the same time) that their problems would have been worse
without religion. It is striking that the relevant distinctions are almost
all related to experiencing support from religion.

3.2. Actual mental health care and religion/worldview

The data mentioned above point out very clearly that religion/world-
view is indeed a very important variable in relation to mental problems. But how is religion/worldview being dealt with in the practice of
therapy?

To start with, it is interesting to look at clients' expectations regarding the attention paid at the Riaggs to questions concerning relig-
ion/worldview. 40% (44%) of the respondents stated to have questions
about religious issues or questions concerning worldview at the assessment interview. 14% (20%) of them strongly expected to receive
help for such questions, 56% (56%) to some degree, and 30% (24%)
expected to get no help at all for such questions. Hence, almost a third
(quarter) of these respondents didn't expect much from the Riagg in
this respect.

How did this materialise in the actual treatment? The following
three questions clarify something of the situation (see Table 3). The
three questions applied to those clients who thought their problems to
be related to religious/worldview issues. The others could tick
'doesn't apply'. The table shows the added percentages of 'fully
agree' and 'partially agree'.

Table 3: *Actual treatment of religious/worldview issues*

		Zwolle/Heerlen
1	At the Riagg there is ample scope for bringing up the religious/worldview aspects of my problems.	61 / 72
2	I had the feeling that the therapist did understand the religious/worldview aspects of my problems.	60 / 62
3	The treatment I've received fitted the religious/world-view aspects of my problems.	36 / 36

There were two more questions about the actual treatment. All respondents, including those who didn't think that there was a relation
between their problems and their religion/worldview, could answer
these questions. 6% (13%) answered that their therapists had asked

about their religious background in a very profound and explicit way; 44% (39%) that they had asked to some degree; 50% (49%) that they had not asked at all.

Of the clients who saw a relation between their problems and their religion/worldview, 13% (25%) answered that their therapists had asked about their religious background in a very profound and explicit way; 59% (51%) to some degree; 29% (24%) not at all.

Of the clients who said that they could not have been treated without having been allowed to talk about their religion/worldview, 17% (29%) answered that their therapists had asked about these issues very profoundly and explicitly; 52% (43%) to some degree; 31% (13%) not at all.

'Did the therapist ever mention a possible referral to a pastor or vicar?', was the second question. 3% (1%) of the clients answered with 'yes', 97% (99%) said 'no'.

How can these figures be understood? Firstly, it appears that it has been possible for clients to talk about religious/worldview issues related to their problems. About 60-70% of clients are satisfied in this respect. A client said: "My therapist is open to my outlook on life and she also respects it, although she doesn't have the same worldview. She admits that she isn't sure whether my point of view is right or wrong. But she is using my worldview in therapy".

Secondly, usually therapists did understand the client's point of view concerning the religious/worldview aspects of the problems. Three out of five of the clients with religious/worldview questions were content with the situation.

Thirdly, at the same time only one out of three was satisfied with the way in which treatment fitted the religious/worldview aspects of their problems. It seems that therapists could, and also wanted to listen to the religious/worldview aspects of the problems, but that they failed to endeavour concrete initiatives in this domain in their therapy. A client stated: "I could talk about the way religion helped me with my problems, but there was no reaction because she wasn't familiar with my religion. I feel very unhappy about that." In this context we can add that most respondents who saw a relation between religion/worldview and their problems replied that their religious background had been discussed only to some degree.

Hardly ever had clients been referred to a pastor or vicar. A client said: "Before I saw my therapist for the first time, I visited Mr X with my husband; Mr X was an official of the ecclesiastical court at that time. When I applied for therapy Mr X said: 'Tell them they can ask me for information about you'. My therapist has never done that! When I asked for an appointment with the priest who worked at the Riagg, my therapist replied: 'Oh that won't be necessary, you have intrapsychic problems'."

A last question in this section was: Was it important to you to be treated by a therapist with the same religion/worldview as yourself? The answers were given as follows:

- yes, very important: 10% (8%)
- yes (to some degree):   14% (10%)
- no, not really: 28% (29%)
- no, it didn't matter at all: 49% (53%)

Especially older people found this important. Of the people of fifty years and older, 23% (20%) placed great importance on allocation to a therapist with the same religion/worldview (total group of respondents 10%). One client said: "When you are dealing with an institution like the Riagg, and you try to live as a good Christian yourself, it's good to find a therapist who feels the same way. Or at least, people who are not indifferent or hostile to it."

Of course there were also correlations with variables that measured various aspects of religiosity. For those to whom religion meant a lot, who believed in a personal God and attended church often, it was more important to be treated by a therapist who had the same religious outlook on life. Regarding the various religious denominations, the differences were striking: for example 'very important' was the reply of:

- 0% of Roman Catholics
- 12% of Dutch Reformed
- 24% of Calvinists
- 14% of other denominations
- 3% of non-religious people.

(Again the figures apply for Zwolle only).

Most respondents however (80% (85%)) didn't know if they had been treated by a therapist with the same religion/worldview. 4% (7%) had been treated by a therapist with the same religion/worldview, 16% (8%) has not been treated by a therapist with the same religion/world-view. From the 51 respondents who placed great importance on the fact that the therapist had the same religion/worldview, only 12 did get such a therapist, 12 didn't get such a therapist, and 27 didn't know if the therapist had the same religion/worldview.

3.3. Wishes of the respondents regarding the role of religion/world-view in their treatment

Evaluation of the actual treatment can best be implemented against the background of the clients' wishes. To what extent do they want religious/worldview aspects to be dealt with in therapy at the Riagg? We have collected the following data. First, we present the data of the group of clients who had no questions regarding their religion/worldview (Table 4). Then we present the data of the group of clients who had questions regarding their religion/worldview (Table 5). The percentages apply to the clients who agree or partially agree.

The majority of those who had no questions regarding religious/worldview issues from the start, did not feel the need to talk about these issues with a therapist familiar with religion/worldview. Referral to a priest/minister was not under discussion. That doesn't imply that they disagreed with the notion that talking about religion/worldview can be most advisable in Riagg therapy for other clients. The majority felt that therapists should be trained to deal with religious aspects of problems and also felt that treatment of this kind of problems belongs to the jurisdiction of the Riagg. The majority felt no need to call in the help of a priest or minister with respect to religion/worldview.

Table 4: *Wishes with regard to religion/worldview in therapy (respondents without questions regarding religious issues)*

		Zwolle/Heerlen
1	During their training Riagg therapists should learn how to deal with religious/worldview aspects of problems.	72 / 62
2	A priest or minister is more capable of dealing with problems related to religion/worldview.	28 / 25
3	I can be treated just as well without talking about my religion/worldview.	72 / 79
4	It is important to me to get a therapist familiar with my religion/worldview.	25 / 26
5	It is important to me to get a therapist of the same religion/worldview.	12 / 06
6	I wanted to be referred to a priest or minister.	05 / 03

Table 5: *Wishes with regard to religion/worldview in therapy*
(respondents with questions regarding religious issues)

		Zwolle/Heerlen
1	During their training Riagg therapists should learn how to deal with religious/worldview aspects of problems.	86 / 82
2	A priest or minister is more capable of dealing with problems related to religion/worldview.	26 / 16
3	I can be treated just as well without talking about my religion/worldview.	34 / 51
4	It is important to me to get a therapist familiar with my religion/worldview.	58 / 54
5	It is important to me to get a therapist of the same religion/worldview.	38 / 31
6	I wanted to be referred to a priest or minister.	23 / 18

The majority of those respondents who had (some) questions concerning religious/worldview issues from the start, also agreed with the opinion that these issues belong to the jurisdiction of the Riagg. Therapists should be trained in dealing with religious issues and again, these clients felt no need to call in the help of a priest or minister. With respect to their own treatment or therapy, almost 60% (54%) placed importance on getting a therapist familiar with their religion/worldview. 40% (31 %) would have liked to have had a therapist of the same religion/worldview. 23% (18%) wished (to some degree) for referral to a priest or minister. But also a third (half) was of the opinion that it wasn't necessary to introduce religion/worldview in the process of therapy.

Further analysis shows that especially respondents, who had experienced a positive influence of their religion/worldview on their problems, wanted a referral to a priest or minister. Probably people are not eager to discuss negative experiences with religion/worldview with a priest or minister.

4. Recommendations

What do these results mean for a policy aiming at improving the quality of treatment with respect to religion and worldview? We will give an answer following five recommendations made by the former manager of the Zwolle Riagg in a volume of symposium proceedings entitled 'Worldview and the Riagg: past, present and future' (Dost 1992, 18).

1   'Questions about religion, worldview and meaning of life should be discussed by psychotherapists themselves'. To achieve this, workshops (for instance lasting at least one half day) should be planned. Important topics for such a workshop could be:
    (a) How do psychotherapists manage their own religion and worldview? Insight is needed, in order to be able to avoid undesirable countertransference reactions (Kerssemakers 1989).
    (b) How can, in the process of treatment, religion and worldview be dealt with in a methodologically appropriate way? To what extent are religious interventions allowed? What to think of the recommendations by some authors in the United States (Lea 1982), to pray and read the Bible together with clients in whose lives religion plays an important role?

2   'The dialogue between the fields of mental health care and pastoral care should be initiated or continued. Pastoral workers should become involved in the process of referring clients.' This involvement should not only apply to the referral of clients to mental health care by clergy, but also to the referral of clients to clergy by psychotherapists. Our research has shown that the latter hardly occurs. Apart from referring, this dialogue could also be applied to mutual consultation and discussion. In this respect, initiatives that have already been taken to bring clergy in contact with psychotherapists could be continued. These meetings have shown that both professions maintain a lot of stereotypes about each other's work and competence. The Zwolle Riagg has organised successful follow-up meetings. Psychotherapists and clergy now have more realistic ideas about each other's work and promising contacts have evolved.

3   'In every Riagg members of staff have to be appointed, with as a special task to cover the area of religion and worldview. They should be accessible to both mental health workers and clergy.' Several Riaggs in the Netherlands now have appointed such a person. Our research data have shown that especially in the Zwolle region the religious backgrounds of the respondents are very differentiated. The above-mentioned 'religious specialists' should be acquainted with the faith communities and religious/philosophical sects and groups in the region. They have to know about these groups' ideas about religion/worldview on the one hand, and how

they think about mental health and mental health care institutions on the other hand. The Zwolle Riagg already uses such an overview or map of groups (especially Protestant denominations are covered) (Vellenga 1992). There is, however, always the risk that this specialist position becomes an alibi for the other mental health workers. They too should develop knowledge and attitudes regarding therapeutic interventions on the one hand and religion/worldview on the other hand. The support for knowledge increase and attitude change should be as broad as possible. Financial resources have to be found to make this possible.

4 'The Riaggs' policy regarding attention for religion and worldview should be supported by empirical research'. The results of the research project reported here is only a starting point. The relation between religion/worldview and mental problems should now be investigated in-depth by means of interviews. We also need an inventory (through review of literature and empirical research) of the experiences of psychotherapists regarding their interventions in the treatment of religious clients.

5 'Initiatives of individual Riaggs should be co-ordinated and supported at a national level.' As stated, there is a growing interest in studying the relations between religion/worldview and health care, in particular mental health care. We can point at the activities of:
 – The Christian College 'Windesheim' in Zwolle;
 – The Zwolle and Heerlen Riaggs;
 – The Radboud University Nijmegen;
 – The Catholic Study Centre for Public Mental Health in Tilburg.
But co-ordination and financial support at a national level are not yet to be found. That is why new initiatives have to be taken.

References

Bauduin, D. (red.) (1991) *Herzuiling in de GGZ? Meningen en discussie over de relatie tussen levensbeschouwing en geestelijke gezondheidszorg in de jaren negentig ['Re-Pillarisation' in Mental Health Care? Opinions and Debates about the Relationship between Worldview and Mental Health Care in the Nineties].* Utrecht: NcGv.

Dijkhuis, J.H. & Mooren, J.H.M. (1988) *Psychotherapie en levensbeschouwing [Psychotherapy and Worldview].* Baarn: Ambo.

Dost, A.J. (1992). Riagg en levensbeschouwing. Een persoonlijke ervaring [Riagg and Worldview: A Personal Experience]. In: Damen, E., Wurff, van der A. & Aberson, J. *Levensbeschouwing en de Riagg. Verleden, heden en toekomst [Worldviews and Riagg. Past, Present and Future].* Zwolle: Riagg-Zwolle.

Draak, den C. (1990) *Lezing kennismakingsbijeenkomst Riagg-Zwolle – Geestelijke Verzorgers regio Zwolle op 19 februari en 19 maart 1990 [Presentation at Introductory Meeting of Riagg Zwolle and Zwolle Area Chaplains, 19 February and 19 March 1990].* Zwolle: Hogeschool Windesheim/Riagg-Zwolle.

Draak, den C. & Kleingeld, K. (1991) *Levensbeschouwing in het welzijnswerk. Verslag van een praktijkgericht onderzoek naar de rol van levensbeschouwing bij bestuurs- en direktieleden, uitvoerend werkers en cliënten van twee confessionele instellingen voor welzijnswerk [Worldviews in Welfare Work. Report on a Practice-Oriented Investigation of the Role of Worldviews in Board and Executive Members, Staff and Clients of Two Confessional Welfare Work Agencies].* Zwolle: Studiecentrum Welzijnswerk en Levensbeschouwing Windesheim.

Easton, A. (1990) *Bejaardenoorden en levensbeschouwing. Deel 1: Begripsbepaling, beleid en thematische uitwerkingen [Homes for the Elderly and Worldview. Vol. 1: Concepts, Policies and Thematic Elaborations].* Amstelveen: Algemene Vereniging van Instellingen voor Bejaardenzorg.

Filius, R. & Visch, M. (eds.) (1991) *Zin in welzijn. Over levensbeschouwing en professionaliteit in het welzijnswerk [Meaning in Well-Being. About Worldview and Professionality in Welfare Work].* Zwolle: Studiecentrum Welzijnswerk en Levensbeschouwing Windesheim.

Groen, de I. & Slockers-Beverwijk, G. (1987) *Religie en psychotherapie. Literatuuronderzoek en een onderzoek op twee Riagg's. Doctoraalscriptie vakgroep klinische psychologie, Rijksuniversiteit Leiden. [Religion and Psychotherapy. Literature Review and an Investigation in Two Riaggs. 'Doctoraal' Dissertation Dept. of Clinical Psychology, State University Leiden].*

Kerssemakers, J.H.N. (1989) *Psychotherapeuten en religie. Een verkennend onderzoek naar tegenoverdracht bij religieuze problematiek [Psychotherapists and Religion. An Exploratory Study of Countertransference with Respect to Religious Problems].* Nijmegen: Katholiek Studiecentrum.

Lans, van der J., Pieper, J. & Uden, van M. (1993) Levensbeschouwing en geloof in de geestelijke gezondheidszorg. Een onderzoek onder Riagghulpverleners [Worldview and Faith in Mental Health Care. An Investigation among Riagg Staff]. *Psyche & Geloof 4*, 111-125.

Lea, G. (1982) Religion, Mental Health and Clinical Issues. *Journal of Religion and Mental Health 21*, 336-351.

Molenkamp, R. (1994) Depressief of troosteloos, een belangrijk onderscheid [Depressed or Disconsolate, an Important Distinction]. *Zin in Welzijn 5*, 2-5.

Nvagg. (1989). *Inventarisatie met betrekking tot cliënten van gereformeerde gezindte [Stock-Taking with Respect to Clients from the Reformed Denomination]*. Interne nota. Utrecht.

Nvagg. (1990). *Verslag onderzoek kwaliteitsbeleid Riagg's [Report on a Study of Riaggs' Policies regarding Quality]*. Utrecht.

Pieper, J.Z.T. & Uden, van M.H.F. (1993*a*) *Ex-cliënten over de Riagg-OZL. Resultaten van een satisfactieonderzoek onder cliënten van wie de behandeling bij de Riagg-OZL te Heerlen in 1991 is afgesloten [Former Clients about the Riagg-OZL. Results of a Satisfaction Survey among Clients whose Treatment in the Riagg-OZL in Heerlen has been Completed in 1991]*. Heerlen: Universiteit voor Theologie en Pastoraat.

Pieper, J.Z.T. & Uden, van M.H.F. (1993*b*) *Ex-cliënten over de Riagg Zwolle. Resultaten van een satisfactieonderzoek onder cliënten van wie de behandeling bij de Riagg Zwolle in 1991 is afgesloten [Former Clients about the Riagg Zwolle. Results of a Satisfaction Survey among Clients whose Treatment in the Riagg Zwolle has been Completed in 1991]*. Heerlen: Universiteit voor Theologie en Pastoraat.

Riagg en religie (landelijke werkgroep) (1991) *Beleidsnota 'Riagg en religie' [Riagg and Religion (National Task Force) (1991) Policy Document 'Riagg and Religion']*.

Schilder, A. (1987) *Hulpeloos, maar schuldig. Het verband tussen een gereformeerde paradox en depressie [Helpless Yet Guilty. The Connection between a Reformed Paradox and Depression]*. Kampen: Kok.

Schilder, A. (1991*a*) Eigen over- of ongevoeligheden t.a.v. een christelijke levensbeschouwing [Our Own Hypersensitivities or Insensitivities towards a Christian Worldview]. In: Filius, R. & Visch, M. (eds.) *Zin in Welzijn. Over levensbeschouwing en professionaliteit in het welzijnswerk. [Meaning in Well-Being. About Worldview and Professionality in Welfare Work]*. Zwolle: Studiecentrum Welzijnswerk en Levensbeschouwing Windesheim, 41-49.

Schilder, A. (1991*b*) Overtuiging, hulpverlening en verslaving [Belief, Help and Addiction]. *Zin in Welzijn 2*, 12-14.

Schilder, A., Schippers, A. (1990) *Religie in therapie [Religion within Therapy]*. Kampen: Kok.

Vellenga, S.J. (1992) *Zin, ziel, zorg. Over levensbeschouwing en geestelijke gezondheidszorg [Meaning, Soul, Care. On Worldview and Mental Health Care]*. Kampen: Kok.

Visch, M. (red.) (1991) *Leven beschouwen en hulp verlenen [Worldview and Helping]*. Zwolle: SWL-Windesheim publ.

Wal, van der J. (1991) *Principes en praxis van gereformeerde hulpverlening [Principles and Practice of Reformed Mental Health Care]*. Lezing op studiemiddag 'Riagg en geloof'. Tiel.

CHAPTER 3

RELIGION IN MENTAL HEALTH CARE: PSYCHOTHERAPISTS' VIEWS

1. Introduction

In a review of ten years (1984-1994) of research on religion and psychotherapy, Worthington *et al.* (1996) indicate that since 1986 the interest in religion and counselling has been booming (see also Worthington 1986).

As we said in chapter 2, in the last few years in the Netherlands the interest in the relation between meaning, worldview and religion on the one hand and social and mental health care on the other hand, is growing too. First we pointed at a series of recent publications on the topic. Moreover, there were a growing number of conferences on this relation. Furthermore, several documents about policies and strategies for managing these issues in the mental health care institutions have been published.

In an earlier publication (Van Uden & Pieper 1996) we have discussed five ways in which psychotherapists may be confronted with religious aspects in their clients' mental problems.

1. Some authors emphasise that excesses in religious socialisation cause or continue mental problems.
2. It is also possible that religious socialisation is conducive to a religion that can function as a healing power. Without religion the mental problems would have been more serious.
3. Thirdly it is also possible that mental problems are on the contrary connected with the absence of religious socialisation. The secularisation process in Western society means that churches and other institutions that used to transmit systems of meaning have lost their influence. Hence, psychotherapists are confronted with clients (especially young people) who experience a loss of meaning and who are not able to frame their life in a comprehensive worldview.
4. In the fourth way the connection goes the other way around: from mental problems to religion. Intrusive life crises, especially those

connected with physical and mental suffering, lead to asking questions like: 'why me?', 'why do these things happen specifically to
me?', 'what did I do?', 'why is this my fate?'. In these situations
people try to get control over their problems by attributing causal-
ity as well as meaning to them (Bulman & Wortman 1977). The
sources of these attributions can be found in religion and worldview.

5. A last way religion can be encountered in therapy has to do with
the change of Western industrial states into multicultural societies.
Psychotherapists meet with a growing number of clients who have
been raised in countries with a non-Christian tradition, in particular
clients with an Islamic background (Kortmann et al. 1993).

2. Religion and psychotherapists

What does this mean for the practice of mental health care in the regional community mental health care institutions in the Netherlands,
called Riaggs. As stated earlier in chapter 2 we have found two central
premises. In the first place there is agreement that religion and worldview could and should have a prominent place in many psychotherapeutic interventions. The physical, emotional, behavioural and social
problems that the clients bring in, are often related to their systems of
meaning and their religious attitudes. In the second place, and simul-
taneously, psychotherapists are being accused of neglecting this dimension. Some, especially those who are close to the Protestant tradition, are in particular concerned about the religious values of the clients (Schilder 1991a; 1991b; Van der Wal 1991). In the latter group
there are also authors who argue that clergy should be working in the
institutions for regional community mental health care, and there are
even authors who advocate founding new regional community mental
health care institutions, based on Christian principles; the Gliagg is an
example of such an institution.

Representatives of the Riaggs however disagree with this last as-
sertion. They state that even in highly religious regions in the Netherlands there are enough Riagg therapists with sufficient expertise regarding the religious backgrounds of the clients.

3. Empirical evidence

The arguments discussed above regarding the practice of psychotherapy are predominantly based on personal experiences, but are these experiences representative for the Riaggs in general?

Because of the lack of empirical evidence we started a research-project in 1992 among Riagg clients (Pieper & Van Uden 1996a; 1996b; see also chapter 2).

In this investigation we used the concepts 'worldview' and 'religion' and they were defined as follows. 'When we speak of worldview we refer to the whole of values, standards and ideas people use when thinking of the meaning and purpose of life. We speak of religion when these values, standards and ideas, as a whole or in part, derive from an existing religious institution (for instance Roman Catholicism or Protestantism).' For most people who have participated in our study, their worldview is a religious one.

Our main conclusions were:
- in about 40% of cases religion/worldview had had a positive influence on mental problems;
- in about 35% of cases religion/worldview had had a negative influence on mental problems;
- religion/worldview could be the cause of problems, while at the same time having healing effects on these problems;
- for most clients there was ample scope for bringing up religious/worldview aspects of their problems, they also felt that the therapists did understand the religious/worldview aspects of their problems, but only 36% of the clients was satisfied with the actual treatment of these religious/worldview aspects;
- there were hardly ever contacts between therapists and clergy;
- especially older people and people belonging to a Calvinist denomination place importance on being treated by a therapist from their own denomination.

But these are the clients' opinions. How do therapists evaluate the place of religion/worldview in therapy? To get an answer we started in 1996 a pilot-study among therapists of two Riaggs in the South of the Netherlands. We also sent the same questionnaire to the therapists of the aforementioned Gliagg. The questions in the questionnaires we sent to them were targeting four main areas or topics.
1. The religious/worldview backgrounds of the therapists.
2. The relation of religion/worldview to mental problems: did the

therapists think there is any relation, and if so, is this a positive and/or negative one?

3. We also asked about the ways therapists had reacted to these relig-ious/worldview dimensions of mental problems: were these prob-lems dealt with as relevant to the therapy or were they avoided, and what kind of religious therapeutic interventions were used?

4. What kind of contacts did exist between therapists and clergy?

In this chapter (see also: Pieper & Van Uden 1997a, 1997b) we will concentrate on the results from the investigation among Riagg thera-pists, but we will also refer to some results obtained from Gliagg therapists. This could clarify in what ways Riagg therapists differ from Gliagg therapists in managing religious components of their cli-ents' problems.

4. Results

4.1. Response rate and characteristics of the therapists

We contacted 134 therapists from two Riaggs in the South of the Netherlands. 65 of them participated in the research, i.e. a return rate of 49%. We have some evidence (through discussions with therapists and staff) that therapists with a favourable view of religion were over represented. The average age of the response group was 42.5 years. Women and men were equally represented. 20% of them worked with youth, 60% with adults and 20% with older people. The main thera-peutic affiliations were: behavioural (25%), social psychiatric ap-proaches (22%) and client-centered therapy (19%).

In the Gliagg we contacted 38 therapists of whom 29 participated, i.e. a return rate of 76%.

4.2. Religious/worldview backgrounds of the therapists

The first part of the questionnaire dealt with the therapists' religious/ worldview backgrounds.

Religious socialisation and present religiosity
The majority of the psychotherapists had had a religious socialisation (70% answered 'yes' and 23% answered 'somewhat'). In the Gliagg

all of the therapists said they had had a religious socialisation.

The present religiosity of the Riagg therapists however showed that only half of the therapists believed in the existence of God (45% agreed, 40% disagreed and 15% couldn't choose).

35% of the therapists were members of a church or religious congregation, 52% were not and 12% couldn't make up their minds. Of the Dutch population at large, 40-60% (on this point various studies disagree) are members of a church or religious congregation.

3% of the therapists attend church weekly. For the general Dutch population (figures 1996), this is 21% (Dekker *et al.* 1997).

100 % of the Gliagg therapists are church members. All of them attend church at least once a week.

Saliency of religion/worldview
There were also questions about the saliency of religion/worldview. How important is religion/worldview to their daily lives? The replies to the next five statements (see Table 1) give the answer. Between brackets we present the scores for the Gliagg therapists.

Table 1: *Importance of religion/worldview to daily life (%)*

	totally agree	agree	nor agree, nor dis-agree	dis-agree	totally dis-agree	never thought about
My religion/worldview is of great importance to my political views.	11 (28)	31 (55)	14 (10)	35 (3)	8 (0)	1 (3)
Without my religion/worldview, my life would look completely different.	11 (45)	28 (52)	25 (3)	26 (0)	6 (0)	5 (0)
When making important decisions, my religion/worldview plays a decisive role.	12 (62)	38 (38)	25 (0)	20 (0)	5 (0)	0 (0)
I am very much interested in religion/worldview.	12 (62)	40 (35)	29 (3)	15 (0)	3 (0)	0 (0)
My religion/worldview is of great importance to my daily life.	17 (59)	40 (38)	26 (3)	17 (0)	0 (0)	0 (0)

About half of the Riagg respondents indicated that religion/worldview was of great importance for their lives.

For the Gliagg respondents' religion/worldview was of great importance in almost all aspects of daily life.

4.3. Relations between religion/worldview and mental problems

The second part of the questionnaire dealt with the relation between religion/worldview and mental problems. How often do the therapists see a relation between these areas?

On the average the Riagg therapists did find such a relation in 18% of their clients. In the Gliagg the therapists did see such a relation in 67% of their clients.

The Riagg therapists, who saw a relation, saw as often a positive influence of religion/worldview as a negative influence.

Negative influence
Let us first look at the kinds of negative relations encountered. 46 out of 65 therapists (71%) did sometimes see clients in their practices, for whom religion had a negative influence. How did this negative influence manifest itself? In Table 2 we present several kinds of negative influences and at the same time indicate how often these negative influences occurred according to the therapists.

Table 2: *Negative influence (%)*

	often	sometimes	never
Religion/worldview emphasises guilt and feelings of guilt.	67 (25)	26 (68)	7 (7)
Clients hold conflicting values, standards and ideals.	50 (19)	48 (70)	2 (11)
Religion/worldview emphasises values like humility, servitude and sacrifice.	43 (28)	50 (61)	7 (11)
Religion/worldview affects people's autonomy.	33 (3)	59 (66)	9 (31)
Clients have a negative outlook on life and future life.	39 (24)	44 (69)	17 (7)
Clients have lost a orienting religion/worldview.	28 (11)	57 (78)	15 (11)

A relation between religion and guilt has often been reported in the literature (Freud 1907; Schilder 1987). Our Riagg data support this finding. Two out of three therapists said that they often saw a relation between these two variables. The relation between humility and religion, which also has been reported often (Derksen 1994) was less found in psychotherapeutic treatment. 43% of therapists reported that they often saw this relationship in their practices.

In the Gliagg too the relation most often reported was the one between religion and guilt. The relation least often reported in the Gliagg had to do with the way in which religion affects autonomy. Only 3% of the Gliagg therapists thought that religion often had a negative influence because it affects people's autonomy.

Positive influence
46 of 65 Riagg therapists (71%) did meet in their practice with clients for whom religion had a positive influence. How did this positive influence manifest itself? In Table 3 we present several kinds of positive influences and we also indicate how often these kinds of positive influences occurred according to the Riagg therapists.

Table 3: *Positive influence (%)*

	often	sometimes	never
Religious rituals provide something to hold on to.	62 (46)	30 (46)	8 (7)
Religion/worldview creates meaning.	54 (93)	44 (7)	2 (0)
Religion/worldview offers security.	41 (82)	59 (18)	0 (0)
Fellow-believers provide social support.	26 (71)	68 (29)	6 (0)
You can consult a pastor.	17 (50)	78 (50)	4 (0)

According to the Riagg therapists, religious rituals were the most influential positive factor (religious rituals provide something to hold on to: 62%). The Gliagg therapists rated this as the least influential factor: 46%.

Next were the religious cognitions (religion/worldview creates meaning: 54%). According to the Gliagg therapists, this was the most influential factor: 93%.

Third in line was the religious feeling of security: 41%. The religious community was attributed with the least positive influence: support from fellow-believers and support from a pastor scored only 26%

respectively 17%. Of the Gliagg therapists, 71% often saw a positive influence because of the social support provided by fellow-believers.

Kinds of mental problems and influence of religion/worldview
The next question was: are there special mental problems in which the influence (both positive and negative) of religion/worldview is particularly present or absent? First we examined the relation between types of problems and positive influence. Ten mental problems were presented and the therapists should choose those problems in which the positive influence was particularly evident. 56 therapists (86%) answered this question. The results are listed in Table 4.

Table 4: *Positive influence in relation to type of mental problem (%)*

	Riagg	(Gliagg)
Experiences of loss	95	(100)
Traumatic experiences	50	(68)
Identity crises	32	(40)
Depression	27	(36)
Anxiety, phobic complaints	25	(44)
Guilt, moral dilemmas	23	(36)
Being a victim of incest	11	(44)
Psychosis	11	(16)
Sexual and relational problems	9	(40)
Anorexia/bulimia	4	(21)

Experiences of loss were by far most often connected with a positive influence of religion/worldview. We have already seen that Riagg therapists in particular connected positive influence with religious rituals. Combining these two findings could mean that religion/worldview had its most positive influence in offering religious rituals, like burial, in order to cope with the death of a loved one.

In two areas most of the Gliagg respondents too saw a positive relation with religion/worldview: experiences of loss and traumatic experiences. Religion functioned as a coping mechanism in times of crisis for both groups of respondents.

The same question was asked with regard to negative influence. The results are listed below in Table 5.

Table 5: *Negative influence in relation to type of mental problem (%)*

	Riagg	(Gliagg)
Guilt, moral dilemmas	82	(64)
Sexual and relational problems	75	(48)
Depression	67	(76)
Identity crises	51	(24)
Being a victim of incest	46	(86)
Psychosis	40	(32)
Traumatic experiences	39	(36)
Anxiety, phobic complaints	39	(36)
Anorexia/bulimia	17	(24)
Experiences of loss	14	(16)

Three kinds of problems were mentioned by more than two out of three Riagg therapists: guilt, sexual and relational problems and depression. All these problems possibly referred to the strict moral codes common in Christian denominations in the decades after the Second World War.

In the view of the Gliagg therapists, guilt, depression and incest were in the top three. Consequently, Riagg therapists as well as Gliagg therapists mention guilt and depression most frequently as mental problems in which a negative influence of religion is particularly present.

4.4. Treatment of religious/worldview aspects of mental problems

The third category of questions dealt with the actual treatment of religious/worldview aspects of mental problems. What kinds of therapeutic interventions do we encounter in the therapeutic practice of the respondents?

Assessment phase
During the exploratory interview or at the beginning of treatment 28% of Riagg therapists regularly asked questions about the religious backgrounds of the clients. 31% did this sometimes and 41% never did.

All of the Gliagg therapists asked questions about the religious backgrounds of their clients.

Case conferences
During case conferences with colleagues, religious/worldview aspects of mental problems were 'sometimes' discussed in 77% of cases, in 22% of cases 'never' and in 2% of cases 'often'. Hardly ever were these discussions profound.

In the Gliagg this was done more often and more profound, according to the therapists.

Actual treatment
48 of the 65 respondents (74%) indicated that they treated clients whose problems included aspects of religion/worldview. In almost all cases (98%) the therapists examined the way in which religion *functioned* in their clients' lives. The great majority (87%) also examined the *content* of religion/worldview.

Table 6: *Religious interventions (%)*

	often	sometimes	never
I go into the client's religious/worldview background.	23 (66)	69 (34)	8 (0)
I use religious/worldview language.	17 (59)	52 (38)	31 (3)
I confront the client with the religious/worldview values of his tradition.	8 (14)	69 (83)	23 (3)
I use so-called leave-taking rituals.	12 (0)	56 (52)	31 (48)
I refer to biblical persons, stories and symbols.	4 (41)	54 (51)	42 (7)
I involve the religious congregation for support.	2 (24)	58 (72)	40 (3)
I bring up my own religious/worldview experiences.	4 (3)	50 (38)	46 (59)
I recommend participating in religious/worldview activities.	2 (28)	44 (62)	54 (10)
I use religious/worldview literature.	4 (35)	35 (62)	60 (3)
I use religious rituals.	0 (0)	27 (14)	73 (86)
I recommend to forgive someone.	0 (0)	21 (10)	79 (90)
I myself forgive the client.	2 (4)	13 (14)	85 (82)
I pray privately for the client.	2 (41)	13 (55)	85 (3)
I pray with the client.	0 (0)	6 (21)	94 (79)
I use Bible drama.	0 (0)	6 (14)	94 (86)
I read the Bible together with the client.	0 (0)	4 (35)	96 (65)

Of the Gliagg therapists, 100% treated clients with religious/world-view problems and examined content and function of religion/world-view.

Did the therapists in dealing with religious/worldview aspects use counselling techniques of a religious nature? 16 of such techniques were presented and the therapists had to indicate whether they 'often', 'sometimes' or 'never' used these techniques. Table 6 shows the results. The techniques are ordered according to the extent that they were used (1= 'often'; 2= 'sometimes' and 3= 'never').

Most religious techniques were used sparingly. The only more or less accepted technique was going into the client's religious/world-view background.

The Gliagg therapists, apart from going into their client's religious background, also said they often used religious/worldview language and prayed privately for the client.

4.5. Competence with regard to religion/worldview

Did the Riagg therapists have enough skills at their disposal for treating religious/worldview aspects of mental problems? Asked for their own opinion, 34% (82% Gliagg) said 'yes', 34% (4% Gliagg) said 'no' and 32% (14% Gliagg) couldn't make up their minds. Some groups of therapists were more confident about their competencies than others. Men were more confident than women: 47% against 19%. Also, those over 34 years old were more confident than those under 35 years: 40% against 12%.

Therapists thought that the skills their colleagues had in this area were more or less equivalent to their own. 12% indicated that their colleagues had enough skills at their disposal, 14% thought they didn't have enough skills. But here we found a much larger group that replied 'I don't know'. 74% was uncertain about their colleagues' skills. (At the Gliagg 82% thought that the skills of their colleagues equalled their own.)

In summary: of the Riagg therapists that could make up their minds, half agreed and half disagreed with the statement that therapists had enough skills at their disposal for treating religious/world-view aspects. At the Gliagg a great majority thought they had enough skills at their disposal. Did this lead to a need for more training in this area? 46% of the therapists felt this need, the other half didn't. Here too some groups deviated from the average. Women and therapists under 35 years of age (both groups with relatively low confidence in this area) felt a more than average need for more training: 59% respectively 63%. Yet two other groups have to be mentioned: therapists working with older people (58% of them felt a need for more training) and client-centered counsellors (75% of them felt a need for more training). Surprisingly, also 57% of the Gliagg therapists still felt a need for more training.

4.6. Contacts with clergy and spiritual directors

The fourth and last part of the questionnaire dealt with contacts between therapists and clergy or spiritual directors (see also Meylink & Gorsuch 1988). The first three questions related to contacts with clergy/spiritual directors in the region, regarding the *actual treatment of clients* having mental problems including religious/worldview aspects. What kinds of contacts did exist? Table 7 shows the results.

Table 7: *Contacts with clergy or spiritual directors regarding actual treatment of clients (%)*

	often	sometimes	never	I don't treat such clients
Regarding these clients, do you contact clergy or spiritual directors in order to support actual treatment?	0 (10)	37 (86)	48 (3)	15 (0)
Regarding these clients, do you ask clergy's or spiritual directors' advice?	0 (7)	25 (72)	60 (21)	15 (0)
Do you refer these clients to clergy or a spiritual counsellor?	0 (28)	46 (72)	39 (0)	15 (0)

The contacts were rather few. Referral to clergy or spiritual directors happens in 46% of cases 'sometimes'. But when we asked how many clients really had been referred, this turned out to be the case with only 1.3% of clients.

According to the Gliagg therapists, these contacts were substantial. Referral (28%) had the highest score. In 6.3% of cases this had actually taken place.

Next, we presented six *more general* statements about contacts with clergy or spiritual directors. The therapists had to indicate whether they agreed or disagreed with these statements. Table 8 shows the results. The statements are presented in decreasing order of importance.

Table 8: *Contacts with clergy or spiritual directors (%)*

	agree	don't know	disagree
Actually I don't have any contacts with clergy or spiritual directors in the region where I work.	69 (14)	0 (3)	31 (83)
As far as I'm concerned, more contacts between psychotherapists and clergy or spiritual directors are not necessary.	34 (17)	47 (24)	19 (59)
Our institution should, in its policy, opt for regular consultations with clergy and spiritual directors in the region.	23 (46)	46 (14)	31 (39)
Actually I don't know how to refer clients with religious/worldview aspects in their mental problems to clergy or spiritual directors.	17 (3)	13 (0)	70 (97)
Clients with religious/worldview aspects in their mental problems are in good hands with the clergy and spiritual directors of the region.	15 (48)	80 (45)	5 (7)
Actually I have no confidence in the competencies of the clergy or spiritual directors in the region.	8 (3)	54 (28)	38 (69)

Most therapists knew how to refer clients to clergy or spiritual directors (70%). Those who were members of a church most easily knew how to refer. The therapists themselves had rather few contacts (31%) with clergy or spiritual directors. Here also those who belonged to a church had the most contacts (48%).

Because of these few contacts it was no surprise that many therapists had no opinion about the competencies ('in good hands' and 'confidence in the competencies') of the clergy or spiritual directors: we found 80% en 54% 'don't know'-scores. Those who had an opinion, had confidence in the competencies of clergy and spiritual directors.

With regard to improvement and intensification of the contacts (more contacts and more consultations), the opinions were divided: about 20% agreed, about 30% disagreed and about 50% had no opinion.

Almost all of the Gliagg therapists knew how to contact the clergy. Their confidence in their competencies was high. But there was also a substantial group (45%) that had some doubts regarding the question whether clients with religious/worldview aspects in their mental problems were in good hands with the clergy.

5. Conclusions

Let us summarise the main conclusions.
1. With regard to the religious backgrounds of the therapists the following conclusion can be drawn. Compared with Dutch citizens in general, therapists believed less in God and had a lower rate of weekly church attendance. The response rate of 49% is also an indication that the research topic was not that interesting to the therapists of the two non-denominational Riaggs (see also Bergin & Jensen 1990; Ragan et al. 1980).

   For the Gliagg therapists, faith was a fundamental value. They all believed in God and went to church at least once a week.
2. With regard to the relation between religion/worldview and mental problems, the following conclusions can be made. 40% of the clients reported a relationship between these two variables (see chapter 2). Riagg therapists reported such a relationship for only 18% of their clients.

   The Gliagg therapists reported this relationship for 67% of their clients. With regard to the kind of relationship, we can conclude that clients pointed more to the positive influence of religion/ worldview than did Riagg therapists.

   Of the Riagg therapists who saw a relation, half of them saw a positive relation, half of them a negative one. The Gliagg therapists on the other hand pointed more to the positive influence of faith.

   For the Riagg therapists, the negative influence was especially connected with guilt, sexual problems and depression. The positive influence was especially connected with the function of religious rituals in coping with experiences of loss and trauma.

   For the Gliagg therapists, the negative influence had to do with the ways in which religion emphasises feelings of guilt and humility and creates a negative outlook on life and feelings of depression.

   On the positive side the Gliagg therapists pointed at religion's function of offering meaning and security, as well as at the social support it provides in dealing with experiences of loss and trauma.

3. With regard to the actual treatment of religious/worldview aspects of mental problems, most Riagg therapists said that they explored these aspects. At the same time, however, half of them did not feel confident about their skills for treating these aspects, and this led to a need for more training (46%). Specific religious techniques were hardly used.

All Gliagg therapists said they dealt with the religious/world-view aspects of mental problems and that they used several relig-ious techniques. 41% of them prayed privately for clients. 80% felt confident about their skills in dealing with religious problems. Yet, 57% would like more training in this area.

4. Contacts between Riagg therapists and clergy were rather few. Re-ferral occurred in only about 1% of cases. This absence of contacts was probably not due to a lack of confidence in clergy, but rather to a fairly complete separation between the worlds of the therapists and the clergy.

In the Gliagg the contacts were substantial. The Gliagg thera-pists knew how to contact the clergy and had confidence in their competencies.

5. Combining these conclusions, we can say that the religious dimen-sion in Riagg psychotherapy could have had a more prominent place. The Gliagg therapists obviously were more open to the relig-ious/worldview aspects of mental problems than were their Riagg colleagues. How this was effectuated in actual practice, however, is still an open question.

Analysing results of more qualitative research among several Riagg as well as Gliagg therapists might enable us to conclude in more detail what these quantitative results mean and what kind of nuances should be made.

References

Bergin, A.E., Jensen, J.P. (1990) Religiosity of Psychotherapists. A National Survey. *Psychotherapy 27*, 3-7.

Dekker, G., Hart, de J. & Peters, J. (1997) *GOD in Nederland 1966-1996 [GOD in the Netherlands 1966-1996]*. Amsterdam/Hilversum: Anthos/RKK/KRO.

Derksen H. (1994) *De parel in het zwarte doosje. De rol van het geloof in de psychische problemen van katholieke Limburgse vrouwen [The Pearl in the Black Box. The Role of Faith in the Mental Problems of Roman Catholic Women in Limburg]*. Nijmegen: De Wetenschapswinkel Nijmegen.

Dijkhuis, J.H. & Mooren, J.H.M. (1988) *Psychotherapie en levensbeschouwing [Psychotherapy and Worldview]*. Baarn: Ambo.

Freud, S. (1907) *Zwangshandlungen und Religionsübungen [Obsessive Actions and Religious Practices]*. Freud Studienausgabe, 1975, Band 7, 11-21. Frankfurt: Fischer Verlag.

Meylink, W.D. & Gorsuch, R.L. (1988) Relationship between Clergy and Psychologists. The Empirical Data. *Journal of Psychology and Christianity 7*, 56-72.

Pieper, J.Z.T., Uden, van M.H.F. (1996a) Geloof en levensbeschouwing binnen de Riagg-hulpverlening. Ex-cliënten aan het woord [Faith and Worldview in Riagg Treatment. Former Clients' Views]. *Psyche & geloof. 7*, 115-127.

Pieper, J.Z.T. & Uden, van M.H.F. (1996b) Religion in Mental Health Care. Patients' Views. In: Verhagen, P.J. & Glas, G. (eds.) *Psyche and Faith. Beyond Professionalism*. Zoetermeer: Boekencentrum, 69-83.

Pieper, J.Z.T. & Uden, van M.H.F. (1997a) *Geloof en levensbeschouwing binnen de Gliagg Dordrecht. Houdingen van therapeuten [Faith and Worldview in the Dordrecht Gliagg. Therapists' Attitudes]*. KUN-rapport: Heerlen.

Pieper, J.Z.T. & Uden, van M.H.F. (1997b) *Geloof en levensbeschouwing binnen de Riagg's te Heerlen en Sittard. Houdingen van therapeuten [Faith and Worldview in the Heerlen and Sittard Riaggs. Therapists' Attitudes]*. KUN-rapport: Heerlen.

Ragan, C., Newton Malony, H. & Beit-Hallahmi, B. (1980) Psychologists and religion. Professional Factors and Personal Belief. *Review of Religious Research 21*, 208-217.

Schilder, A. (1987) *Hulpeloos maar schuldig. Het verband tussen een gereformeerde paradox en depressie [Helpless Yet Guilty. The Connection between a Reformed Paradox and Depression]*. Kampen: Kok.

Schilder, A. (1991a) Eigen over- of ongevoeligheden t.a.v. een christelijke levensbeschouwing [Our Own Hypersensitivities or Insensitivities towards a Christian Worldview]. In: Filius, R., Visch, M. (eds.) *Zin in welzijn. Over levensbeschouwing en professionaliteit in het welzijnswerk [Meaning in Well-Being. About Worldview and Professionality in Welfare Work]*. Zwolle: Windesheim, 41-49.

Schilder, A. (1991b) Overtuiging, hulpverlening en verslaving [Belief, Treatment and Addiction]. *Zin in Welzijn 2*, 12-14.

Uden, van M.H.F. & Pieper, J.Z.T. (1996) *Religie in de geestelijke gezondheidszorg [Religion in Mental Health Care]*. Nijmegen: KSGV.

Wal, van der J. (1991) *Principes en praxis van gereformeerde hulpverlening [Principles and Practice of Reformed Mental Health Care]*. Lezing op studiemiddag 'Riagg en geloof'. Tiel.

Worthington E.L. Jr. (1986) Religious counseling: A review of published empirical research. *Journal of Counseling and Development 64*, 421-431.

Worthington, E.L. Jr., Kurusu, T.A., McCullough, M.E. & Sandage, S.J. (1996) Empirical Research on Religion and Psychotherapeutic Processes and Outcomes: A 10-year Review and Research Prospectus. *Psychological Bulletin 119*, 448-478.

CHAPTER 4

PSYCHOTHERAPY AND RELIGIOUS PROBLEMS ILLUSTRATION BY MEANS OF A CASE HISTORY

In the Netherlands, religion and mental health care have grown apart in the process of secularisation. Nowadays however, one can witness a growing need among counsellors and psychotherapists to be educated in the areas of religion, meaning giving and worldviews (Van der Lans *et al.* 1993; Raaijmakers 1994). That religion has returned to the focus of attention, can also be concluded from the fact that in a recent version of the diagnostic bible, the DSM IV, a separate code (code: V 62.89) has been included for religious or spiritual problems (Lukoff *et al.* 1992). The case history of a patient with an obsessive-compulsive disorder that we will present, is meant as a contribution to this educational process. We will show how important it is to look at the religious frame of reference of a patient and how this can be managed in psychotherapeutic treatment. The case will be positioned within the theoretical perspective of symbolic interactionism (Mead 1934).

1. Theoretical notions

According to George Herbert Mead (1934), the self develops in a process of role taking: in interactions, individuals assume the roles, or perspectives, of the other, and evaluate their own behaviour 'through the eyes of the other'. By taking the perspective of the other person, people become self-conscious. They learn to reflect upon themselves as objects. The part of themselves of which people are conscious, is the 'me'; it comprises several self-other systems, corresponding to the important relationships in the different areas of their environments. In this process the individual can take the role of a specific other or of a generalised other. The generalised other represents a group to which an individual belongs or wants to belong. For the development of the self it is very important that people learn to take the role of a generalised other, enabling them to learn to anticipate the expectations and reactions of the group. By internalising these expectations and demands in the 'me', people are able to act in conformity with them. The 'me' represents our adjustment to an organised world. Our ability to take the role of a generalised other makes us relatively independent of specific others in particular situations. The 'me', however, can comprise specific others as well. The 'me' enables us to be members of our society, but it cannot determine the ways in which we behave as social beings. It provides the self with an inner representation of the social structure that limits our actions. The action itself, however, depends on the 'I', i.e. the part of the self that is inaccessible to immediate reflection. The 'I' is the creative, innovating aspect of the self; it gives us a sense of freedom and initiative. It is this unknown aspect of ourselves that we try to realise in our actions. The 'me' constitutes the structure that makes this self-realisation possible.

Mead rejects the view of the self as an independent entity or unit in the person. The 'self' should be understood as a process, as a continuing inner dialogue between two different but connected 'voices': the 'I' and the 'me'. Traces of the 'I' can be found in the form of central themes in the person's life history, as they take shape on the basis of biological urges and early experiences in the interaction with primary others, and as they are enacted throughout one's life in various social roles. Role taking is the process through which people reflect upon themselves and give meaning to their actions and their environment.

Meaning emerges in a process of anticipation and reaction; it depends on a given social structure and on the previous experiences of the individual who imparts meaning.

Meaning, whether implicit in little everyday aspects of life or more explicit in a search for the meaning of life, always emerges from the interaction between the sensitive individual and what comes to them from their environment.

A system of meaning is a cognitive complex of beliefs, attitudes, values and norms that people construct during their personal history in a continuing process of interpretation, systematisation and legitimisation of themselves, others and events, by which people structure themselves as a totality and transcend their immediate life situation, impart meaning to their lives and acquire a relative subjective security.

This individual system of meaning can be regarded as part of the cognitive system of humans. The cognitive system helps the individual to recognise and label experiences. The system of meaning has a specific controlling and integrating function within this cognitive system. Characteristic of this system of meaning is that it deals with 'existential questions', questions that transcend day-to-day experiences.

In correspondence with Mead's conception of the self, the individual system of meaning comprises several self-other systems that are based on the interactions of the self with significant others, and that function as sources of meaning. The sources of meaning that people acquire, and which one they will use, depend on their life-history and the specific situation in which they find themselves. Notwithstanding the fact that people make use of different sources of meaning in different situations, they experience themselves as an unity, as a single person. This is due to the primary self-other system that integrates the many sources of meaning into a totality of meaning, while this in turn is affirmed and given content by the sources of meaning. In accordance with Mead's line of thought, one might stipulate that the sense of unity is due to the 'I'-aspect of the self: the person's identity that they seek to realise through their several self-other systems.

This primary system is constructed through the interaction with a so-called primary other. The relationship of a child with its parents usually influences the primary self-other system more than e.g. relationships with colleagues at work. We therefore make a hierarchical difference between on the one hand the primary self-other system as the most important part within the structuring and integrating system of meaning, and the other self-other systems on the other hand, being domains of life to which the primary self-other system imparts meaning. The important other in the primary self-other system can be a specific person, if, for example, the relationship self-mother structures the total impartment of meaning, or it can be a generalised other, e.g. the family, a social group or community. With respect to developmental psychology, it is important to note that a sound development ranges from relationships with specific others to relationships with generalised others. For further details we refer to Van Uden (1985).

Relevant in this context is the question how to stimulate this process in order to turn a problematic relationship with a primary specific other into a relationship to a primary generalised other that offers perspective. Elsewhere (Van Uden 1988) we have stressed that rituals can fulfil this transforming function and we made clear that in psychotherapy such a ritual transformation can be realised. The patient can be provided with a meaning that fits seamlessly into his process of searching for meaning, and then true meaning can be found. We consider it to be one of the tasks of the clinical psychology of religion to supply ideas and concepts that are helpful in searching for the seamless fit mentioned above. But what does this look like in practice? And which therapeutic interventions can be made? We want to underline here that this requires modesty. Often, minimal, well-timed and well-dosed interventions are needed, in which the theoretical concepts mentioned above can play a guiding role. A generally applicable procedure is not available. In the area of the clinical psychology of religion still more time has to be spent in collecting, describing and analysing psychotherapeutic case histories, in which an evident religious dimension is included in the psychopathology and the treatment process (see also Wikström 1994, 230). In the following section we therefore present the case of Mr Rigstra (see Van Uden 1996).

2. The case of Mr Rigstra

This section will describe the treatment of a man from a strict religious environment, who was severely suffering from obsessive neurotic problems. In the recapitulation we will try to connect the concrete case history to the theoretical concepts discussed previously.

2.1. Initial situation

At the age of 32, Mr Piet Rigstra was referred by the Employment Office for psychotherapy. Mr Rigstra had been unemployed for almost ten years. In the past he had worked for a few months for a contractor and afterwards for various other employers. He had completed primary and secondary school without difficulties and according to his teacher he had the capacity for General Secondary Education. Nevertheless he went to Junior Technical College at his father's insistence, who alluded to their religious beliefs: "Our church tells us not to pursue higher aspirations. Junior Technical College is sufficient and humility is a great good". Hence, Mr Rigstra started Junior Technical College in his hometown. He never passed his finals.

He was the eldest from a family of seven children and came from an Evangelical, religious congregation. Since a few years his father had been the religious leader of this congregation. At home he had received a traditional upbringing, causing him to appear, as he said, old-fashioned. There used to be a content atmosphere at home, which was determined by their faith. At the age of twelve, Mr Rigstra had been "moved by the spirit of God" and at that time, he said, he had been truly happy. He had been married for ten years to a woman of the same religious persuasion and had two children.

His behaviour, at entering therapy as over the past years, was greatly determined by obsessive compulsive neurotic problems, the cause of which lay in a period of time in which he had started to seclude himself more and more. During the first years at Junior Technical College he had been bullied by classmates because of his aberrant religious beliefs and his behaviour that resulted from, among other things, these beliefs. He had tried to temper the accompanying tension through elaborate cognitive obsessive rituals, the effect of which had decreased over time.

2.2. Course of treatment

First three sessions

Mr Rigstra himself considered his current situation to be the result of 'a blow to his nervous system', that he had been struck at Junior Technical College at the time. He had not been able to stick up for himself and had been bullied around. He had become an object of ridicule and pestering. He said that thinking of his Junior Technical College time still made him shiver. When we explored his complaints, they turned out to be an obsessive 'getting stuck'. If he read an article in which certain letters appeared, then these letters reminded him of the names of the bullying boys at Junior Technical College. He had not fitted in with the rest and in the end he had failed his finals twice, distracted as he had been by what he called fretting. It was amazing that he had got married and had children, considering how he actually had filled his days since the age of fifteen. There were hardly any ways for him to relax by reading, watching TV or pursuing hobbies. He had not read for years for fear that he would encounter certain letters that would render him stuck.

Fourth and fifth sessions

In these sessions we tried to get a clear picture of how his obsession was composed. We explored his blocks and discovered the following obsessive system as a remedy for the blocks: 'If something gets stuck in my thoughts in a conversation, I grow restless, which will only get less if I repeat it twice in my mind for five times. Then an additional seven times, and at the fifth time of this third set of repetitions, the tension has gone'. For example, in a conversation it could happen that the words 'oom' and 'laan' were used. These were emotionally charged letter combinations, referring to the names of two boys (Dohmen and Van Laan) from the period of bullying at Junior Technical College. Hearing in particular the vowels 'o' or 'a' was enough to put a block on Mr Rigstra. Neutralising this block was achieved through an extremely complicated cognitive procedure in which three sets of five repetitions played an important role (during which he, additionally, softly humming clenched his teeth). The problem seemed to be bigger than Piet himself realised. It was a cognitive, complex series of linking thoughts. He mentioned that he sometimes did not give in and that this made him feel good. More often, however, he returned, literally, to the place of doom. This was the place where something had got stuck in his mind, e.g. a traffic light, where he had been waiting and had been confronted with certain words or sounds.

Sixth and seventh sessions

During these sessions we paid closer attention to the causes which lay at he bottom of his obsession. Piet understood that an emotionally charged past during the first years of secondary school, over the years had led to the development of generalising obsessive rituals which warded off fear and had spread to larger parts of his life. Furthermore, it became clear to him that a lot of unexpressed anger was hidden in this. Anger which was managed by means of a magical ritual. This ban on being angry was legitimised by religious formulas. Do not return evil with evil, was the message that his father had given him for years. Our reference to Jesus who had chased the merchants from the Temple in a not very gentle way left him silent for a long while and evidently shocked his convictions.

Eighth session

During this session Piet was rather confused. The theme was having 'wrong' thoughts and 'removing' this negativity that caused him headaches. Piet's strategy so far consisted in going to the person about whom he had had a negative thought and asking him to forgive him for having had this thought. It seemed as if in this way, he was ridding himself more and more of his own opinions about matters and people. If an opinion did develop, he nipped it in the bud. His religious convictions helped him to do so: 'Do not think evil of your brothers'.

Ninth and tenth sessions

For the time being the treatment process was focused on 'identity confirmation', by having him express during the sessions what he thought and felt, without masking or denying it. The sessions were now a place to practice saying what he thought without any restraints. Piet said that after the last few sessions he had left singing. For the first time he felt understood. Despite the weight and the extent of his problems, Piet could laugh and loosened up.

Eleventh session

During this session, it was explained to Piet that in order to fight his obsessions, he had to learn to prevent his responses. We agreed that in the next week he would suppress his obsessive inclination about one minor event and would continue his activities, even if the tension increased.

Sessions 12 and 13

Piet mentioned that his 'activities to conquer his obsession' were going fairly well. Moreover, he had allowed his negative opinions while talking to others. Remarkably, during the sessions he was able to speak more fluently. It seemed as if Piet increasingly was breaking free from his isolation. He was considering buying a TV set, for example, and wondered whether, instead of standing at the entrance of his favourite soccer team, he should go inside to watch an entire game, without punishing himself for enjoying the game by leaving before it was over. With regard to his progress, he was asked to keep a diary of his experiences.

Sessions 14, 15, 16, 17 and 18

Piet wanted to broaden his horizon but gradually ran into problems concerning his religious background. "How can I learn to enjoy to be free if my religion (personified in his father) weekly dins into me that all enjoyment will lead me astray from the narrow path to the Lord?"

His feeling of guilt about this brought along a need to punish himself. The therapeutic strategy consisted in exposing Piet to situations which were burdening to him, by means of an 'exposure procedure', starting with less burdening situations and forbidding him to use rituals to settle his feelings of guilt. Writing down his progress, however, was very laborious, because too many words with 'wrong' vowels had to be written down. Writing the letters 'o' and 'a' always confronted him with stress, and looking back at it required too much effort. As a solution he deformed all letters, thus considerably diminishing the legibility.

Sessions 19, 20, 21, 22, 23, 24 and 25
Piet focussed on his writing, but continued to get stuck. He could not put away his notebook after he has finished writing. We agreed that he would ask his wife to check that he, while writing at home, did not pay more than five minutes to this 'reading aftercare'. Nevertheless, it became clear that Piet had to struggle tremendously in order to keep going. His tension obviously was increasing. In various areas Piet reported stagnation and problems in getting started.

Sessions 26, 27 and 28
In a reckless mood Piet had tried to read the newspaper for the first time in years, with disastrous results. For hours he had had to practice his ritual in order to relieve the tension built up. We decided that next time he would bring along a newspaper page and that we would systematically go into his reading problems.

Sessions 29, 30, 31 and 32
When tackling his problem reading the newspaper, it turned out that he was especially bothered by the large number of separate columns of text having numerous burdening letters in the headlines. While reading (...) the bottom left of the page, his eyes wandered off to different places, where he incidentally saw the word 'doorgaan', for example. Knowing that this burdening word was there then made it impossible for him to put away the newspaper without having practised the ritual for a long while. During the following sessions all kinds of strategies were used to tackle this 'big size' problem. By cutting the newspapers into pieces, increasingly larger pieces of newspaper were presented to him. Repeatedly it was evident that Piet could only stop if

the amount of text was limited to a few lines. This stagnation in progress demoralised Piet considerably.

Sessions 33, 34 and 35
The 'reading improvement strategies' continued to go up and down. We decided to leave the newspaper articles for the time being and to focus on books. The advantage of a book turned out to be the limited letter space. Thinking about the question which book would be most suitable, we suggested the Bible. "Yes", Piet said, "if only I could read my father's book." We agreed that from now on he would daily read to his children from the Bible. Furthermore, we suggested that he – of course – could not treat the Bible – being the word of God – as disrespectful as the newspaper. The Bible as a holy book ought not to be abused for his compulsive ritual. This message turned out to catch on miraculously. Piet Rigstra was able to read without practising his compulsive ritual. He was proud of himself and said that finally he felt that he was a father to his children. Every night at a set time he read to his family. "At last I can really mean something to them."

Sessions 36, 37, 38 until end of treatment
Many more sessions were to follow, in which the benefits achieved at this level could gradually be transmitted to other parts of life. Piet engaged, for example, more explicitly into discussions with his own father, during which he was able to express what he felt and to do what he wanted. In various areas he breached his father's strict standards. It was obvious that this also loosened his tie with his religious congregation. Nevertheless, it was to be expected that the job that he found after termination of treatment as well as his marriage would provide sufficient structure to replace the until now safe yet oppressing function of the religious group run by his father.

2.3. Recapitulation

How did the various therapeutic interventions achieve what they did? The psychotherapeutic process is, among other things, meant to optimise dispositions to change and to estimate which ingredients will enable a change. It is of crucial importance that, apart from using the 'technique', a link is made with what earlier in this contribution was called the 'primary self-other system'. In the case of Mr Rigstra's treatment, alongside the obvious behaviour therapeutic approach, two aspects from the religious domain have been of great importance in his process of change: (a) expressing aggression without apologies, sanctioned by the image of the infuriated Jesus in the Temple; (b) reading aloud from his father's book, the Bible, with the idea of it being a 'holy book' helping him not to give in to his compulsive ritual.

In both cases he was having a dispute with his father. In the first case he put aside his father's ban on aggression with the help of the higher religious authority of Jesus (represented by the authority of the therapist!). In the second case he took the role of father upon himself in the eyes of his children and partner by reading to them, something which had not happened for years. Moreover, the conviction of not being allowed to abuse the Bible as the word of God helped him to control his obsession. Thus the religious domain in Mr Rigstra's life not only had a repressive side but it also offered some beneficial means. In Mr Rigstra's case we can say that, with respect to the effectiveness of the 'religious interventions', put in terms of the theoretical frame of thought described previously, these interventions fitted in with his 'primary self-other' structure. Through these interventions a beginning has been made with the development of breaking free from the all-determining relationship with the 'primary specific other': father. If the psychotherapeutic process succeeds in fitting in with the primary structure, as happened in this case, finding meaning can occur and the patient is freed of his galling bonds with the primary specific other. This process requires imagination and inspiration. It is possible that this inspiration can only be found if patient and psychotherapist together enter the illusional world and 'intermediate sphere' of which Pruyser (1992) and Winnicott (1971) speak. This inspiration cannot be planned or learned: it requires an attitude of openness. Schachtel (1959) would call it an allocentric perception. Then it can suddenly become clear that a linking-line connecting God, father and Bible can have a therapeutic effect. We see this kind of insight as a form of finding meaning. We hope with the presentation of the case of Mr Rigstra to have provided a glance into the treatment room of the clinical psychologist of religion.

3. Conclusion

Mr Rigstra's case can serve to add the following considerations regarding education and training of counsellors and psychotherapists. Through this case we have wanted to show how complex the role of religion is in the individual's psyche. Even in an a-religious (often even antireligious) psychotherapeutic approach like behaviour therapy, attention paid to religion and meaning can be of great importance.

In general the training of counsellors and psychotherapists leaves hardly any room for paying attention to this dimension of existence. What, then, is possible and necessary in the regular training courses, with regard to this issue? In our opinion, during such courses, psychotherapists should at least have explored their own religious/existential past. If this has not happened, even an unbiased reflection on the role of religion in therapy is hardly possible, let alone interventions with a positive effect. Counsellors and psychotherapists should be able to talk about meaning and religion, and to listen to their clients' religious backgrounds. This would require a client-centered approach. Preferably, they also should have a large number of stories, rituals and symbols from the Christian tradition at their disposal. However, in order not to indoctrinate, they should be able not only to re-evaluate this tradition in the framework of present-day time and culture (Lukken 1988), but also to apply it to their clients' personal settings. This can only be done in an adequate manner if they know themselves in regard to this religious/existential dimension. An important aid would be a training course in which psychotherapists and counsellors are taught to deal with their own religious/existential pasts in such a way that it will not be an obstacle to understanding others. Technically speaking, they would have to learn how to manage professionally their countertransference reactions in the area of religion. Only by knowing our own beliefs, we can truly discern other people's beliefs.

References

Freud, S. (1907) *Zwangshandlungen und Religionsübungen [Obsessive Actions and Religious Practices]*. Freud Studienausgabe, 1975, Band 7, 11-21. Frankfurt: Fischer Verlag.

Kerssemakers, J.H.N. (1989) *Psychotherapeuten en religie. Een verkennend onderzoek naar tegenoverdracht bij religieuze problematiek [Psychothe-*

rapists and Religion. An Exploratory Study of Countertransference with Respect to Religious Problems]. Nijmegen: Katholiek Studiecentrum.

Lans, van der J., Pieper, J. & Uden, van M. (1993) Levensbeschouwing en geloof in de geestelijke gezondheidszorg. Een onderzoek onder Riagg-hulpverleners [Worldview and Faith in Mental Health Care. An Investigation among Riagg Staff]. *Psyche & Geloof 4*, 111-125.

Lukken, G. (1988) *Geen leven zonder rituelen [No Life without Rituals]*. Baarn: Ambo.

Lukoff, D., Lu, F. & Turner, R. (1992) Toward a More Culturally Sensitive DSM-IV. Psychoreligious and Psychospiritual Problems. *The Journal of Nervous and Mental Disease 180*, 673-682.

Mead, G.H. (1934) *Mind, Self and Society*. Chicago: University of Chicago Press.

Pruyser, P.W. (1992) *Geloof en Verbeelding. Essays over levensbeschouwing en geestelijke gezondheid [Faith and Imagination. Essays on Worldview and Mental Health]*. Baarn: Ambo.

Raaijmakers, C. (1994) *Religie en hulpverlening. Een onderzoek naar de plaats van religie in de hulpverlening van de Riagg Groningen [Religion and Treatment. A Study of the Position of Religion in Riagg Groningen Treatment]* Groningen: Riagg Groningen.

Schachtel, E.G. (1959) *Metamorphosis. On the Development of Affect, Perception and Memory*. New York: Basic Books.

Uden, van M.H.F. (1985) *Religie in de crisis van de rouw. Een exploratief onderzoek d.m.v. diepte-interviews [Religion in the Crisis of Mourning. An Exploratory Study by Means of Depth Interviews]*. Nijmegen: Dekker & van de Vegt.

Uden, van M. (1988) *Rouw, religie en ritueel [Mourning, Religion and Ritual]*. Baarn: Ambo.

Uden, van M.H.F. (1996) *Tussen zingeving en zinvinding. Onderweg in de klinische godsdienstpsychologie [Between Imparting Meaning and Finding Meaning. En Route in the Clinical Psychology of Religion]*. Tilburg: Tilburg University Press.

Wikström, O (1994) Psychotic (A-)Theism? The Cognitive Dilemmas of Two Psychiatric Episodes. In: Corveleyn, J. & Hutsebaut, D. (eds.) *Belief and Unbelief. Psychological Perspectives*. Amsterdam/Atlanta: Rodopi, 219-232.

Winnicott, D.W. (1971) *Playing and Reality*. New York: Tavistock.

CHAPTER 5

RELIGIOUS COPING IN TWO SAMPLES OF PSYCHIATRIC INPATIENTS

1. Introduction

As the psychology of religion developed at the end of the nineteenth century, the relation between religion and mental health already was a main topic. James, Hall, Leuba and Starbuck studied questions like: 'Is conversion a sign of pathology or is it on the contrary an attempt to integrate an unstable self?', and 'To what degree are intense religious and mystical experiences connected with mental health and to what degree with psychopathology?' Recent empirical studies suggest "that religious commitment may play a beneficial role in preventing mental and physical illness, improving how people cope with mental and physical illness, and facilitating recovery from illness" (Matthews *et al.* 1998, 118).

In line with this tradition, we have been studying for about a decade the influence of religion on the lives of people suffering from mental health problems. Because of the lack of empirical evidence in the Netherlands regarding this question, we started a research project among outpatients in 1992 (see chapter 2; Pieper & Van Uden 1993*a*; 1993*b*; 1993*c*, Van Uden & Pieper 1996). We studied several groups of outpatients. At that time we were in particular interested in the degree of positive versus negative influence of religion on mental problems. Our main conclusions were: in about 40% of cases religion has a positive influence on mental problems; in about 35% of cases religion has a negative influence on mental problems. The positive influence could be understood in line of Pargament's religious coping theory (Pargament 1997). For religious persons in times of mental crisis religion is a powerful tool for managing this crisis. Other authors have come to similar conclusions. "Religion may serve as a pervasive and potentially effective method of coping for persons with mental illness, thus warranting its integration into psychiatric and psychological practice" (Tepper *et al.* 2001, 660). Fitchett *et al.* (1997) found that a large majority of the psychiatric patients they studied turned to religion during hospitalisation. Kirov *et al.* (1998) found that about 60% of the psychotic inpatients they studied used religion to cope with their disorder.

In this chapter we will present some results of two new studies. In the first study we investigated a population of moderately religious psychiatric inpatients (sample I), in the second study our respondents were highly religious psychiatric inpatients (sample II). In these studies we focused on three main questions:

1. *To what degree did patients practise religious coping activities?*
   Religion was (very) salient for the investigated samples, so we expected high levels of religious coping, in sample II even more so than in sample I.

2. *To what degree were religious coping activities beneficial to the patients' well-being?*
   Most studies signal positive effect of religious coping on psychological and existential well-being. Pargament *et al.* (2001, 510) studied religious coping of clergy, elders and members of the Presbyterian Church. They concluded that 'religion has more significant effects for those whose roles and identities are more closely tied to religion'. Hence, we expected more positive influence of religious coping on existential and psychological well-being for the highly religious population compared with the moderately religious population of psychiatric inpatients.

3. *To what degree was well-being influenced by the general religiosity of the inpatients and to what degree by their specific religious coping activities?*
   With respect to this question, Pargament *et al.* (1990; 1992) and Jenkins & Pargament (1995) have argued that for the resolution of specific life events, in this study being hospitalised in a mental hospital, situation-specific measures of religiousness should be stronger predictors than generalised measures of religiousness. They have proposed a model of religious coping efforts as mediators of the relationship between general religious orientations and the outcomes of specific life situations. Religion comes to life in immediate stressful life situations. Other researchers though (Fabricatore *et al.* 2000) have pointed at the positive effects of general religiousness (like the perception of a close relationship with God) on well-being, whereby it is not necessary that this general religiousness is transposed into specific religious coping behaviours and

strategies tied to negative life events. Most research (Schaefer & Gorsuch 1991; Park & Cohen 1993; Pargament *et al.* 2000) has concluded that both general religiousness and religious coping contributed significantly and uniquely to the variance in well-being, and that neither was totally eliminated by the other. We also expected to find influences of both general religiousness and religious coping.

2. Method

2.1. Characteristics of the samples

In December 1999 we studied patients of a large-scale mental hospital in the south of the Netherlands: sample I. As research-technique we used questionnaires. 411 patients were addressed. 141 questionnaires were returned. This means a response rate of 34.3%. The age of the participants ranged from 17 to 78 years with a mean of 43 years (n= 137). The median was 44 years. 54% was male, 46% female (n= 138). Because of the low response rate we did a small non-response-investigation. We did expect that people with a positive attitude towards religion and pastoral care are over-represented. Indeed, to some degree this effect occurred. Especially those patients that wanted to contact a pastoral counsellor participated in the investigation. Also those people that experienced a positive influence of religion on their mental problems were over-represented. This means that in the total population the positive influence of religion was not as high as in the response-group.

In December 2000 we investigated patients of a Protestant mental hospital in the central part of the Netherlands: sample II. This hospital has been founded in order to treat patients with an orthodox Reformed (Calvinist branch of Dutch Protestantism) religious identity. For these patients, the central doctrines of their religion are guidelines for their behaviour in daily life, and consequently also for their daily life in hospital. Praying, reading the Bible, church attendance and discussing religious topics is part of the daily routine. The professional staff also has to subscribe to the central doctrines of Reformed Protestantism. As research technique we used questionnaires. All 249 patients treated in the second half of 2000 received a questionnaire. 118 questionnaires were returned. This means a response rate of 47.4%. No non-response research was carried out. The age of the participants ranged from 18 to 79 years with a mean of 39 years (n= 115). The median was 37 years. 54% was male, 46% female (n= 116).

2.2. Religious characteristics of the samples

The majority of the patients of sample I had been religiously social-ised: 69% answered 'yes' and 20% answered 'somewhat', only 11% answered 'no' (n= 139).

In their present life 63% of the patients were member of a religious congregation, 31% were not and 6% couldn't make up their minds (n= 140). A recent sociological study showed (Dekker et al. 1997, 12) that of Dutch citizens in general 47% were member of a church or relig-ious congregation. The vast majority of the church members were member of the Roman Catholic Church: 92%, 6% were member of a Protestant denomination, 1% were Muslim and 1% Jew.

56% of the respondents did sometimes attend church or other relig-ious ceremonies: 15% of the patients went to church weekly, 10% once a month, and 31% only a few times a year. 44% never attended church (n= 141). Of the average Dutch citizen only 40% never at-tended church (Dekker et al. 1997, 14).

How often was one involved in private religious activities like prayer, meditation and reading the bible? 36% were regularly involved in these activities: 11% were involved several times a day, 17% al-most every day and 8% regularly. 22% were sometimes involved in these private religious activities, and 42% were seldom or never in-volved (n= 141). Especially church members were regularly involved in these activities (Chi^2= 32.756; df= 4; s.n.: 0.000). 50% of them were regularly involved in these activities, of the non-church members only 12% were regularly involved.

We used a short version of Hoge's (1972) original Intrinsic-Religiosity Scale to measure the degree of intrinsic religiosity. This is the Duke Religion Index (Koenig et al. 1997), consisting of three items. To be intrinsically religious means that one lives his religion, and that one not uses religion for other ends (Allport 1950; Allport & Ross 1967). About 50% of the respondents agreed with these items, 18% neither agreed nor disagreed, 32% disagreed.

In summary: most of the respondents had had a religious socialisa-tion; over 60% were members of a religious congregation, mostly the

Roman Catholic Church. Half of the patients were intrinsically motivated. However only a quarter regularly attended religious services and only one third was regularly involved in private religious activities. So most of the respondents were religious, but rather in a passive way. This sample was a little more religious than the average Dutch citizen.

The majority of the patients of sample II hade been religiously socialised in childhood: 91% answered 'yes' and 6% answered 'somewhat'; only 3% answered 'no' (n= 117).

In their present life, 97% of the patients were members of a religious congregation, 2% were not and 1% couldn't make up their minds (n= 118). 63% were Reformed (Calvinist branch of Dutch Protestantism) and 35% were Dutch Reformed (Lutheran branch of Dutch Protestantism).

97% of the respondents did attend church or other religious ceremonies: 61% went to church twice weekly, 31% once a week, 3% once a month, and 2% only a few times a year. 3% never attended church (n= 118).

How often were these patients involved in private religious activities like prayer, meditation and reading the Bible? 92% were regularly involved in these activities: 50% were involved several times a day, 17% almost every day and 25% regularly. 7% were sometimes involved in these private religious activities, and 1% seldom or never (n= 118).

Here too we used a short version of Hoge's (1972) original Intrinsic-Religiosity Scale to measure the degree of intrinsic religiosity. This is the Duke Religion Index (Koenig *et al.* 1997), consisting of three items. About 70% of the respondents agreed with these items, 20% neither agreed nor disagreed and 10% disagreed (n= 115).

In summary: almost all of the respondents had had a religious socialisation; over 97% were members of a religious congregation, two out of three were Reformed and one out of three was Dutch Reformed. 70% of the patients were intrinsically motivated. 92% regularly attended religious services and about 90% were regularly involved in private religious activities. Consequently, in comparison with Dutch citizens in general this was a highly religious sample.

2.3. Measures

2.3.1. Religious coping: Pargament's three coping styles

Pargament *et al.* (1988) referred to three ways in which people can deal with issues of responsibility and control in religious coping activities: self-directing, deferring and collaborative. In the self-directing style it is the individual's responsibility to solve problems. The individual takes an active problem-solving stance. In the deferring style, individuals defer the responsibility of problem-solving to God. They wait for solutions to emerge through God's active efforts. In the collaborative style, responsibility for the problem-solving process is held jointly by the individual and God. Both are working together to solve problems.

   Pargament *et al.* (1988) developed a questionnaire to measure these coping styles. The short version of this questionnaire was translated into Dutch by Alma (1998). A few of Pargament's statements had to be reformulated because of differences between the American and the Dutch contexts. This translation has also been used in our research. The questionnaire consists of 18 statements, six statements for each coping style. The response categories are: 1= 'never'; 2= 'seldom'; 3= 'occasionally'; 4= 'often'; 5= 'always'.

2.3.2. Religious coping: additional information

Pargaments's coping styles represent different kinds of problem-focused coping. In our questionnaire we also tried to measure religious coping in another way. We didn't focus on problem-solving, but instead we focused on enduring the situation and managing the emotional distress that is associated with it, for instance by giving meaning to it and looking for social support. Theoretically, the effectiveness of religious coping activities could be summarized briefly as follows: they establish social integration and support; they establish a personal relationship to a divine other; they provide systems of meaning and existential coherence; and finally they promote specific patterns of religious activity and personal life style (Daaleman 1999). Thus, social, affective, cognitive and behavioural aspects are involved. These four aspects were operationalised as follows:

Social aspect:
- My religion has a positive influence on my mental problems because of the support of fellow believers.
- My religion has a positive influence on my problems because I can visit a pastoral counsellor.

Affective aspect:
- My religion has a positive influence on my mental problems due to my relationship with God: I am not on my own.
- My religion has a positive influence on my mental problems because it offers me security.

Cognitive aspect:
- My religion has a positive influence on my mental problems because it provides meaning.

Behavioural aspect:
- My religion has a positive influence on my mental problems because religious rituals, like praying and attending church, provide something to hold on to.
- My religion has a positive influence because prayer and meditation help me to cope with my mental problems.

The response categories were: 1= 'yes', 2= 'somewhat', and 3= 'no'. We have to emphasize that this measure only provides information about successful religious coping.

2.3.3. Spiritual well-being

In this study we used the 'Spiritual Well-Being Scale' (SWBS) to further explore the relation between religion, religious coping and existential and psychological well-being. Paloutzian and Ellison have developed the SWBS noting that there had been little attention for the spiritual and existential aspects of people's lives as a quality of life indicator (Scott *et al.* 1998). The scale consists of two dimensions: a vertical dimension, assessing one's relationship to God (the Religious WBS) and a more horizontal dimension, assessing life purpose and meaning in life (the Existential WBS). Ten statements measure each dimension. However, a study among psychiatric inpatients by Scott *et al.* (1998), using factor analysis, found that for this population a three factor solution with sixteen items was adequate. In our study we used these sixteen items. The American studies used a six-point Likert Scale for answering the statements, we used a five-point Likert Scale, because most of the other scales in the questionnaire were five-point Likert Scales. The patients could give the following answers: 1= 'strongly agree'; 2= 'agree'; 3= 'neither agree nor disagree'; 4= 'disagree'; 5= 'strongly disagree'.

2.3.4. Psychological well-being

Psychological well-being was measured with a psychological scale, the ZBV. The ZBV is a self-examination questionnaire, which is used to determine the amount of anxiety present. This questionnaire is the Dutch version of the STAI, Spielbergers 'State-Trait Anxiety Inventory' (Van der Ploeg *et al.* 1980). The ZBV consists of two separate questionnaires with which two distinct concepts of anxiety can be measured: state anxiety and trait anxiety. As we were interested in long term effects rather than in short term ones, we chose for the Trait Anxiety Scale. This scale is consists of twenty statements like 'I feel fine' and 'I feel nervous and agitated'. Ten statements are symptomatically positive and ten are symptomatically negative in formulation. The alternatives for answering are: 'hardly ever', 'sometimes', 'often' and 'nearly always'. One can score 1, 2, 3, or 4 points per item. Thus the range of the entire scale runs from 20 to 80 points. The lower the score, the lower the trait anxiety.

3. Results

3.1. Spiritual well-being

Before answering our main questions we first have to report upon some preliminary analyses we have done regarding the Spiritual Well-Being Scale. Statements indicating religious and existential well-being were more often endorsed than statements indicating religious and existential doubts. The overall score of the scale underlined this: 2.74 for the mixed religiously sample I and 2.61 for the highly religious sample II (negatively worded items are scored inversely).

The next step in the data analysis of the spiritual well-being scores was an exploratory factor analysis. Was the three-factor solution of Scott, Agresti and Fitchett also recognisable in our data? This was the case for the first sample, but not for the second.

Sample I
We performed a principle component analysis with oblimin rotation; missing pairwise; mineigen= 1; explained variance: 65.8% (40.7%, 17.3% and 7.8%) en KMO (Kaiser-Meyer-Olkin measure for sample adequacy)= 0.88. We found the same three factors as Scott *et al.* (1998).

The first factor, named 'affiliation', consisting of 7 items, indicates a positive affective relationship with God which adds to the sense of well-being. In this factor also a statement with a negative relation with God is included, but this statement has a negative factor-loading. Factor 2, labelled 'existential crisis', consisting of 6 items, indicates a negative existential outlook on life. The only item with a positive outlook on life also is included but with a negative factor-loading. Factor 3 was labelled 'alienation'. The three items of this factor indicate a distance from God. This factor solution differs a bit from the original idea of a religious and an existential part of the SWBS. The existential part is according to the theory, but the religious part is broken into two distinct factors. This means that alienation and affiliation are not exactly two ends of the same continuum.

These three factors were used as scales. The mean of the first scale 'affiliation' (alpha= 0.93) was 2.83. The mean of the second scale 'existential crisis' (alpha= 0.85) was 3.34. The mean of the third scale 'alienation' (alpha= 0.65) was 3.33. This means that a small majority of the inpatients had a positive relationship with God, wasn't in an existential crisis and was not alienated from God. Correlations for each pair of scales were moderately high. The correlation between 'affiliation' and 'existential crisis' was minus 0.34. Consequently, when one had a positive relation with God one was at the same time less in an existential crisis. The correlation between 'affiliation' and 'alienation' was minus 0.56. So, the more positive the relation with God, the less one was alienated from God. The correlation between 'alienation' and 'existential crisis' was 0.41. So, when one had a negative relation with God one was at the same time more in an existential crisis.

In this study we used the 'affiliation scale' as measure of general religiousness, as measure of the inpatients' religious resources. We used the 'existential crisis-scale' as a measure of existential well-being. Low scores on this scale indicate existential well-being.

Sample II
We performed a principle component analysis with varimax rotation; missing pairwise; mineigen= 1; explained variance: 54.8% (43.2% and 11.6%) en KMO (Kaiser-Meyer-Olkin measure for sample adequacy)= 0.88. We found two factors.

The first factor, named 'positive relationship with God', consisting of nine items, indicates a positive affective relationship with God that adds to the sense of well-being ('affiliation'). In this factor also three statements indicating a negative relationship with God ('alienation') are included, but these statements have a negative factor loading. Factor 2, labelled 'existential crisis', consisting of seven items, indicates a negative existential outlook on life. The only item with a positive outlook on life also is included, however with a negative factor loading. This factor also contains the item 'I don't have a personally satisfying relationship with God'. Theoretically, we expected this item to belong to factor 1, but with a negative factor loading. This factor solution differs from the solution of Scott *et al.*, but is in accordance with the original idea of a religious and an existential part of the SWBS.

These two factors were used as scales. But we excluded from the second scale the item 'I don't have a personally satisfying relationship with God'. The mean of the first scale 'positive relationship with God' (alpha= 0.87) was 2.17. The mean of the second scale 'existential crisis' (alpha= 0.83) was 3.31. This means that a majority of the inpatients had a positive relationship with God and was not in an existential crisis. The correlation between 'affiliation' and 'existential crisis' was minus 0.62. Consequently, when one had a positive relationship with God, one was at the same time less in an existential crisis.

In this study we used the 'affiliation scale' as measure of general religiousness, as measure of the inpatients' religious resources. We used the 'existential crisis scale' as a measure of existential well-being. Low scores on this scale indicate existential well-being.

3.2. Religious coping: Pargaments' three coping styles

This measure was only used in the second study: sample II.

From a confirming factor analysis it appeared that the theoretically expected three styles could be distinguished. But two items did not end up in the factors. The two items ('when I feel anxious or nervous about a problem, I search in my prayers together with God for a way to relieve my worries', 'I don't spend much time thinking about troubles I've had; God makes sense of them for me') were removed from the analysis. This led to a factor solution with three factors (principal component analysis with oblimin rotation; missing pairwise; factors= 3; explained variance: 39.7% + 11.1% + 8.6% = 59.4%; KMO= 0.87).

From these three factors, scales were constructed with reliable alphas of 0.87, 0.77 and 0.81 respectively. The collaborative scale scored highest with 3.15, followed by the self-directing scale (2.60) and the deferring scale (2.56). In general, the scores on these problem-focused styles were not high. The patients used them at best 'occasionally'. Some patients told us that they didn't like to talk about God as a problem solver.

From Pargament's study it appeared that the styles are interconnected. This study, too, showed a clear correlation. There was a positive correlation of 0.46 between the deferring and collaborative styles. In both styles, God played an important role. The self-directing style contrasted with the other two styles: with the deferring style (r= −0.43), but even more so with the collaborative style (r= −0.63).

The coping styles were connected with the following social and religious characteristics. The self-directing style occurred less frequently in intrinsic believers (r= −0.54), patients who had a positive relationship with God (r= −0.63), patients who devoted a great deal of time to private religious activities (r= −0.28) and in the elderly (r= −0.35). The deferring style was seen more frequently among intrinsic believers (r= 0.36) and patients who had a positive relationship with God (r= 0.41). The collaborative style was seen more frequently in intrinsic believers (r= 0.48), patients who had a positive relationship with God (r= 0.62), patients who devoted a great deal of time to private religious activities (r= 0.27) and in the elderly (r= 0.25). Again it became apparent that especially the self-directing and collaborative styles were contrasting styles. Regression analysis showed that especially a positive relationship with God predicted the scores on the coping styles: more collaborative and less self-directing.

3.3. Religious coping: additional information

Sample I
In the next table we show how often the kinds of successful religious coping activities we formulated occurred according to the patients of sample I.

Table 1: *Positive influence because... (%)*

	yes	somewhat	no
My religion provides meaning.	50	27	23
My religion offers security.	41	28	31
One can visit a pastoral counsellor.	47	14	39
Due to my relationship with God I am not on my own.	43	21	36
Religious rituals, like praying and church attendance, give me something to hold on to.	39	27	34
Fellow believers provide support.	35	26	39
Prayer and meditation did help in coping with my problems.	33	22	45

(n= 125-129)

Our data indicate that the most positive influence was exercised by the cognitive dimension of religion (providing meaning): half of the respondents agree. The affective dimension (offering security, relationship with God) was for about 40% of the patients applicable. The social dimension has two aspects. Visiting a pastoral counsellor was for more people (47%) a coping resource than the support of their fellow believers (35%). Religious activities showed the least positive influence, whereby public rituals were more favourite (39%) than private religious activities (33%). But maybe the low score on the last item could have been caused by using the word 'meditation', an activity not common in the Christian tradition. Exploratory factor analysis showed that the seven religious coping activities could be reduced to one factor. They were combined into one scale (alpha= 0.89), called positive religious coping.

Sample II
In the next table we show how often the kinds of successful religious coping activities we formulated occurred according to the patients of sample II.

All alternatives (social, affective, cognitive, and behavioural) clearly applied, with one exception: 'prayer and meditation help me to cope'. This item probably applied less because 'meditation' is not a common practice in Protestantism. For this population religion was very helpful in coping with mental problems. This especially held for the older patients. All these items (except for 'one can visit a pastoral counsellor') were positively correlated with age. Exploratory factor analysis showed that the seven religious coping activities could be reduced to one factor. They were combined into one scale (alpha= 0.86), called positive religious coping.

Table 2: *Positive influence because... (%)*

	yes	somewhat	no
My religion provides meaning.	69	22	10
One can visit a pastoral counsellor.	72	14	14
Religious rituals, like praying and church attendance, give me something to hold on to.	67	26	7
Due to my relationship with God I am not on my own.	62	26	12
Fellow believers provide support.	59	30	10
My religion offers security.	54	31	15
Prayer and meditation did help in coping with my problems.	41	35	24

(n= 113-115)

3.4. Religious coping and existential and psychological well-being

Now we will discuss the relation between religious coping (Pargament's three coping styles and positive religious coping) and well-being (existential well-being and psychological well-being). We will start with existential well-being. In sample I positive religious coping correlated positively with existential well-being (r= 0.44).

In sample II existential well-being especially correlated positively with positive religious coping (r= 0.59), but also with collaborative (r= 0.35) and deferring coping (r= 0.32). Existential well-being was negatively correlated with self-directive coping (r= –0.43). Hence, for this highly religious sample, being able to use their religion for religious coping added significantly to their existential well-being, more as compared to the mixed religiously sample (0.59 versus 0.44). If religion was not involved in coping with the problems (self-directive group), existential well-being decreased.

In sample II (there are no data available for sample I) psychological well-being (amount of anxiety) correlated positively with positive religious coping (r= 0.40) and with collaborative coping (r= 0.23). The correlations with deferring and self-directive coping were not significant. Here also, religious coping added significantly to psychological well-being, but not as much as to existential well-being.

3.5. Religiosity, religious coping and existential and psychological well-being

In this section we will discuss the relations between general religiosity, religious coping and existential and psychological well-being. Are situation-specific measures of religiousness stronger predictors for well-being than generalised measures of religiousness? In this study we answered the question by regressing the general religious variables together with the coping variables (positive religious coping and Pargament's three coping styles) in a simultaneous multiple regression equation on the dependent variables: existential and psychological well-being. Table 3 shows the zero order correlations (bivariate analysis) of the religious variables (general and coping) with existential well-being as well as their standardised regression coefficients (linear regression, method: enter).

Table 3: *General religious characteristics and religious coping as predictors of existential well-being*
(Sample I: n= 141; sample II: n= 118)

	Zero order correlations	Beta (standardised regression coefficients)
Intrinsically religious: sample I	0.33***	0.06 n.s.
Intrinsically religious: sample II	0.52**	0.11 n.s.
Affiliation with God: sample I	0.34***	0.14 n.s.
Affiliation with God: sample II	0.62**	0.39*
Religiously active (praying, reading Bible): I	0.18*	0.08 n.s.
Religiously active (praying, reading Bible): II	0.20*	0.00 n.s.
Church attendance: sample I	0.20*	0.05 n.s.
Church attendance: sample II	0.04 n.s.	0.01 n.s.
Positive religious coping: sample I	0.44***	0.41**
Positive religious coping: sample II	0.59**	0.28*
Self-directive coping: sample II	−0.43**	0.04 n.s.
Deferring coping: sample II	0.32**	0.11 n.s.
Collaborative coping: sample II	0.35**	0.09 n.s.

*$p<0.05$; ** $p<0.01$; *** $p< 0.001$; Sample II: R^2 total= 40%*

The bivariate analysis showed that all the religious variables (except for 'church attendance' in sample II) correlated significantly with existential well-being. We have to remind that in this sample almost everybody attends church at least once a week. Hence, there is little variation in the answers on this variable. Regression analysis however indicated that the best predictors of existential well-being in sample II were 'affiliation with God' and 'positive religious coping'. Consequently, a central general religious characteristic as well as an event related religious coping activity were independent predictors of existential well-being. In the sample of the less religious psychiatric inpatients the best predictor of existential well-being was positive religious coping. For these less religious patients, especially religion as a concrete resource in the coping process added to the general feeling of existential well-being.

The same kind of analysis was now undertaken, with psychological well-being (amount of anxiety) as the dependent variable. There are only data for sample II. Table 4 shows the results.

Table 4: *General religious characteristics and religious coping as predictors of psychological well-being*

	Zero order correlations	Beta (standardised regression coefficients)
Intrinsically religious	0.33**	0.16 n.s.
Affiliation with God	0.35**	0.16 n.s.
Religiously active (praying, reading the Bible)	−0.14 n.s.	−0.28*
Church attendance	0.07 n.s.	0.01 n.s.
Positive religious coping	0.40**	0.29*
Self-directive coping	−0.17 n.s.	0.21 n.s.
Deferring coping	0.18 n.s.	0.05 n.s.
Collaborative coping	0.23*	0.09 n.s.

*$p<0.05$; ** $p<0.01$; R^2 total= 20%*

The bivariate analysis showed that four religious variables correlated significantly with psychological well-being: being intrinsically religious, positive relationship with God, positive religious coping and collaborative coping. These are general religious characteristics as well as coping variables. Regression analysis however showed that, of these variables, only positive religious coping had an independent influence. But there was still another remarkable finding: being religiously active (praying, reading the Bible) had a negative influence on psychological well-being (amount of anxiety). A possible explanation could be that without a positive relationship with God, praying and

Bible reading several times a day would be a kind of obsessive ritual in order to control fear (Freud 1907), without success anyway. Finally, the analysis of sample II showed that 20% of the variance of psychological well-being was explained, whereas religion explained 40% of the variance of existential well-being.

4. Conclusions and recommendations

4.1. Conclusions

The analysis of the data leads to the following conclusions. First, most of the respondents of sample I had a religious socialisation, were member of a religious congregation, but only a minority was involved in private and collective religious activities on a regular basis. Almost all of the respondents of sample II had a religious socialisation, were members of a religious congregation, and were involved in private and collective religious activities on a regular basis. This was a highly religious sample having access to extensive religious resources. Especially 'affiliation with God' was a decisive religious characteristic.

Second, for this population of psychiatric inpatients (as well as sample I as sample II), religion was a major source of coping with their mental problems. This applied in particular to the more emotion-focused religious coping. This conclusion corresponds with Pargament's theoretical notions (1990; 1997) about religious coping and with Koenig's (1990) and Koenig et al.'s (1996) notions about religious coping in later life. Inpatients experienced their life situation as relatively unchangeable. They lacked for problem-focused coping. That's why they had to rely on emotion-focused coping strategies. One of the most powerful emotion-focused coping style was the religious one offering possibilities of creating meaning, relying on God, engaging in private and public religious activities and getting social support from the religious congregation.

Third, if religion helps in coping with mental illness – and in our samples this was very much the case – psychological and especially existential well-being are enhanced. This means that religious coping can reduce the amount of anxiety associated with mental problems, and furthermore, even when this is not the case, it can at least contribute to finding meaning and purpose in life. For the highly religious patients, religious coping was more relevant to their existential well-being than for the group of less religious inpatients. If religion has a high salience to an individual's identity, it is very important to experience that in critical periods of life religion contributes to the enduring of these periods. Otherwise the individual's central values will be at stake.

Fourth, what about the relation between general religious resources, religious coping activities and well-being? Elsewhere, Krause & Tran (1989) have made a distinction between the stress-buffering model and the main-effect model. In the stress-buffering model, religion only influences well-being in the presence of stress. This means that in situations of stress general religion has to be tied in specific ways to the stressor in order to exert influence on well-being. In the main-effect model religiosity exerts a general protective effect regardless of the presence or absence of stress factors. In the study of the moderately religious group of inpatients especially the stress-buffering model gets support. For this group we can conclude that most of our respondents had at least latent religious resources. To the degree that these resources became actualised in coping with mental disorders and hospitalisation, this led up to better existential well-being (no measures of psychological well-being were used). But in our research with highly religious inpatients the findings were more complicated. As to the existential well-being, main effects as well as stress-buffering effects were found. As to the psychological well-being (amount of anxiety), especially stress-buffering effects were found. The best predictors of psychological well-being were indicators of religion that were directly connected to the patient's mental problems (positive religious coping). We think that the differences between these two samples regarding existential well-being can be explained by differences in degree of religiousness: moderate versus high. In our highly religious sample the relationship with God was always a central part of self-reflection. Consequently, in evaluating the meaning of life it was an additional source of existential well-being, apart from religion as a coping mechanism.

Finally, we also found a negative influence of religion on mental health (amount of anxiety). Some inpatients could have used praying and Bible reading as an obsessive-compulsive ritual. Consequently, it is also possible to use negative religious coping techniques (Pargament *et al.* 1998).

4.2. Recommendations

Future research should try to avoid several methodological shortcomings of this study. To start with, we need longitudinal designs, as in this cross-sectional design no causal explanations can be given. One could easily conclude that a positive relationship with God leads to less anxiety, but some respondents (in an open question) also reported that feelings of anxiety and depression led to a decline in their religious feelings. Second, newly developed measures of religious coping can be used (Pargament *et al.* 2000). Third, more objective measures of well-being should be used. Our study relied on a self-report measure. It is possible that the positive correlation between religion, religious coping and especially existential well-being is a matter of self presentation. Maybe it is difficult for religious people to admit that the world could be purposeless and meaningless. Furthermore, it is important to pay attention to the research sample. Differences in the degree of religiousness led to different relations between general religiousness, religious coping and well-being. Consequently, different theories are needed to understand the behaviours of different samples. Finally, we need more fine-tuning between the religious doctrines and experiences of the population under investigation on the one hand and the religious coping instruments on the other hand. Orthodox Christian groups differ from more liberal Christian groups in their perceptions of the relationship between human beings and God, whereas for instance New Age oriented religious groups still have other perceptions of this relationship.

Professional staff in mental hospitals should be aware of the potential beneficial effects of religious coping on well-being for religious patients. This means that assessment and treatment should also include patient's religious resources. Furthermore, they would do well to work together with the hospitals' chaplaincies.

References

Allport, G.W. (1950) *The Individual and his Religion.* New York: Macmillan.

Allport, G.W. & Ross, J.M. (1967) Personal Religious Orientation and Prejudice. *Journal of Personality and Social Psychology 5*, 432-443.

Alma, H.A. (1998) *Identiteit door verbondenheid. Een godsdienstpsychologisch onderzoek naar identificatie en christelijk geloof [Identity through*

Alliance. A Study in the Psychology of Religion on Identification and Christian Faith]. Kampen: Kok.

Daaleman, T.P. (1999) Belief and Subjective Well-Being in Outpatients. *Journal of Religion and Health 38*, 219-227.

Dekker, G., Hart, de J. & Peters, J. (1997) *GOD in Nederland, 1966-1996. [GOD in the Netherlands 1966-1996].* Amsterdam/Hilversum: Anthos/RKK/KRO.

Fabricatore, A.N., Handal, P.J. & Fenzel, L.M. (2000) Personal Spirituality as a Moderator of the Relationship between Stressors and Subjective Well-Being. *Journal of Psychology & Christianity 19*, 221-228.

Fitchett, G., Burton, L.A. & Sivan, A.B. (1997) The Religious Needs and Resources of Psychiatric Inpatients. *The Journal of Nervous and Mental Disease 185*, 320-326.

Freud, S. (1907) *Zwangshandlungen und Religionsübungen [Obsessive Actions and Religious Practices].* Freud Studienausgabe, 1975, Band 7, 11-21. Frankfurt: Fischer Verlag.

Hoge, D.R. (1972) A Validated Intrinsic Religious Motivation Scale. *Journal for the Scientific Study of Religion 11*, 369-376.

Jenkins, R.A. & Pargament, K.I. (1995) Religion and Spirituality as Resources for Coping with Cancer. *Journal of Psychosocial Oncology 13*, 51-74.

Kirov, G., Kemp, P., Kirov, K. & David, A.S. (1998) Religious Faith after Psychotic Illness. *Psychopathology 31*, 234-245.

Koenig, H.G. (1990) Research on Religion and Mental Health in Later Life. A Review and Commentary. *Journal of Geriatric Psychiatry 23*, 23-53.

Koenig, H.G., Larson, D.B. & Matthews, D.A. (1996) Religion and Psychotherapy with Older Adults. *Journal of Geriatric Psychiatry 29*, 155-184.

Koenig, H.G., Parkerson, G.R. Jr. & Meador, K.G. (1997) Religion Index for Psychiatric Research. *American Journal of Psychiatry 153*, 885-886.

Krause, N. & Tran, T.V. (1989) Stress and Religious Involvement among Elderly Black Adults. *Journal of Gerontology. Social Sciences 44*, 4-13.

Matthews, D.A., McCullough, M.E., Larson, D.B., Koenig, H.G., Swyers, J.P. & Greenwold Milano, M. (1998) Religious Commitment and Health Status. A Review of the Research and Implications for Family Medicine. *Archive for Family and Medicine 7*, 118-124.

Pargament, K.I. (1990) God Help Me. Toward a Theoretical Framework of Coping for the Psychology of Religion. *Research in the Social Scientific Study of Religion 2*, 195-224.

Pargament, K.I. (1997) *The Psychology of Religion and Coping. Theory, Research, Practice.* New York: The Guilford Press.

Pargament, K.I., Ensing, D.S., Falgout, K., Olsen, H., Reilly, B., Haitsma, van K. & Warren, R. (1990) God Help Me (I): Religious Coping Efforts as Predictors of the Outcomes to Significant Negative Life Events. *American Journal of Community Psychology 18*, 793-824.

Pargament, K.I., Kennell, J., Hathaway, W., Grevengoed, N., Newman, J. & Jones, W. (1988) Religion and the Problem-Solving Process. Three Styles of Coping. *Journal for the Scientific Study of Religion 27*, 90-104.

Pargament, K.I., Koenig, H.G. & Perez, L.M. (2000) The Many Methods of Religious Coping. Development and Initial Validation of the RCOPE. *Journal of Clinical Psychology 56/4*, 519-543.

Pargament, K.I., Olsen, H., Reilly, B., Falgout, K., Ensing, D.S. & Haitsma, van K. (1992). God Help Me (II): The Relationship of Religious Orientations to Religious Coping with Negative Life Events. *Journal for the Scientific Study of Religion 31*, 504-513.

Pargament, K.I., Tarakeshwar, N., Ellison, C.G. & Wulff, K.M. (2001) Religious Coping among the Religious. The Relationships between Religious Coping and Well-Being in a National Sample of Presbyterian Clergy, Elders and Members. *Journal for the Scientific Study of Religion 40*, 497-513.

Pargament, K.I., Zinnbauer, B.J., Scott, A.B., Butter, E.M., Zerowin, J. & Stanik, P. (1998) Red Flags and Religious Coping. Identifying some Religious Warning Signs among People in Crisis. *Journal of Clinical Psychology 54*, 77-89.

Park, C.L. & Cohen, L.H. (1993) Religious and Non-Religious Coping with the Death of a Friend. *Cognitive Therapy and Research 17*, 561-577.

Pieper, J.Z.T. (2004) Religious Resources of Psychiatric Inpatients. Religious Coping in Highly Religious Inpatients. *Mental Health, Religion and Culture 7/4*, 349-363.

Pieper, J.Z.T. & Uden, van M.H.F. (1993a) *Ex-cliënten over de Riagg-OZL. Resultaten van een satisfactieonderzoek onder cliënten van wie de behandeling bij de Riagg-OZL te Heerlen in 1991 is afgesloten [Former Clients about the Riagg-OZL. Results of a Satisfaction Survey among Clients whose Treatment in the Riagg-OZL in Heerlen has been Completed in 1991].* Heerlen: Universiteit voor Theologie en Pastoraat.

Pieper, J.Z.T. & Uden, van M.H.F. (1993b) *Ex-cliënten over de Riagg Zwolle. Resultaten van een satisfactieonderzoek onder cliënten van wie de behandeling bij de Riagg Zwolle in 1991 is afgesloten [Former Clients about the Riagg Zwolle. Results of a Satisfaction Survey among Clients whose Treatment in the Riagg Zwolle has been Completed in 1991].* Heerlen: Universiteit voor Theologie en Pastoraat.

Pieper, J.Z.T. & Uden, van M.H.F. (1993c) *Tevredenheidsonderzoek ouderen. Ex-cliënten van de afdeling ouderen over de Riagg-OZL [Satisfaction Survey among Elderly. Former Unit for Elderly Clients about the Riagg-OZL].* Heerlen: OZL.

Ploeg, van der H.M., Defares, P.B. & Spielberger, C.D. (1980) *Handleiding bij de Zelf-Beoordelingsvragenlijst [Manual of the Self-Assessment Questionnaire].* Lisse: Swets & Zeitlinger.

Schaefer, C.A. & Gorsuch, R.L. (1992) Situational and Personal Variations in Religious Coping. *Journal for the Scientific Study of Religion 32*, 136-147.

Scott, E.L., Agresti, A.A. & Fitchett, G. (1998) Factor Analysis of the 'Spiritual Well-Being Scale' and its Clinical Utility with Psychiatric Inpatients. *Journal for the Scientific Study of Religion 37*, 314-321.

Tepper, L., Rogers, S.A., Coleman, E.M. & Newton Malony, H. (2001) The Prevalence of Religious Coping among Persons with Persistent Mental Illness. *Psychiatric Services 52*, 660-665.

Uden, van M.H.F. & Pieper, J.Z.T. (1996) *Religie in de geestelijke gezondheidszorg [Religion in Mental Health Care]*. Nijmegen: KSGV.

CHAPTER 6

"WHEN I FIND MYSELF IN TIMES OF TROUBLE..." PARGAMENT'S RELIGIOUS COPING SCALES IN THE NETHERLANDS

1. Introduction

One of the ways of measuring religious coping Pargament discusses in his book *The Psychology of Religion and Coping* (1997), refers to the ways people deal with issues of responsibility and control in religious coping activities. In this context he mentions three styles of religious coping: self-directing, deferring and collaborative. By a coping style is meant: "(…) relatively consistent patterns of coping in response to a variety of situations" (Pargament *et al.* 1988, 91). The styles appear to be related to individuals' images of God and the nature of their relations to God, in particular as to the locus of responsibility for solving problems (with the individual or with God), and the extent to which individuals actively try to find a solution and, while doing so, experience God's support. The three styles of religious coping that Pargament *et al.* (1988) distinguish can be characterised as follows:

1. *Self-Directing*
   Solving the problem is the individuals' responsibility and they make efforts to accomplish this. God gives people scope and opportunity to direct their own lives. The religious frame of reference is hardly used in this coping style; compared to the other two styles there is a much looser connection with traditional religiousness.

2. *Deferring*
   Responsibility rests with God; individuals passively wait to see what possible solutions God will offer. Research carried out by Pargament *et al.* shows that this coping style is connected with a religious orientation in which external rules, convictions and authority are looked for in order to satisfy personal needs.

3. *Collaborative*

Responsibility is shared between God and the individual; both make an active contribution to the solution of problems. Research carried out by Pargament *et al.* (1988) demonstrates that the collaborative style correlates with an individual's religious orientation characterised by a personal relation to God, and in which religion is the paramount and motivating life force.

We applied the scales, developed by Pargament *et al.* (1988) in order to gain insight in these religious coping styles in surveys among members of Protestant churches (ecumenical Protestant, Dutch Reformed and Lutheran) and among patients in an Dutch Reformed psychiatric hospital in the Netherlands. In this chapter we will discuss some of the results of these surveys and compare them with Pargament's results. Furthermore, we will deal with some methodological questions and problems connected with the use of these scales. Finally we will present an attempt to develop an alternative scale: one that may accommodate some of the drawbacks inherent in the use of Pargament's scales.

2. The results of the survey by Alma (1998)

In Alma's survey (1998) the 'Three Styles of Religious Coping Scales' were first of all used to select respondents for interviews. On the basis of the results of the survey carried out by Pargament *et al.* (1988), these coping styles could be expected to correlate with the nature of the individual's relationship with God. Indeed, for Alma's survey, which was centred on entering into a religious relation, the instrument offered the interesting possibility of selecting people who differed as to this aspect.

The comprehensive version of the three scales consists of 36 items (twelve statements for each coping style). However, Pargament *et al.* have developed for each scale an abridged version of six items with a high level of internal consistency and a high rate of correlation with the comprehensive version. This has led to the assumption that the abridged version would be adequate for the limited aim of distinguishing three groups in Alma's sample. The decision to opt for this version of eighteen items in all, was also based on our concern that having to go through 36 strongly similar items would lead to irritation with the respondents. We will return to this concern in a later part of this chapter.

As no validated Dutch version exists of the coping style scales, the statements had to be translated as closely as possible to the original English text. It appeared necessary, however, to formulate some statements differently in order to express the same meaning. For example, the statement 'When considering a difficult situation, God and I work together to think of possible solutions' was rendered through the Dutch equivalent of 'When considering a difficult situation, I put it to God in my prayers in order to think of possible solutions together with Him'. The original English statement finds its origin in the representation of God as the 'personified generalised other' who is involved in one's life, a representation that seems to be more common in the American context than in the Dutch context. Now that the translation places the collaboration with God within the context of prayer, people who do not believe in God's direct involvement in their lives can also empathise with the statement.

While we were constructing the questionnaire, we also made an attempt to find a criterion in relation to the question whether or not the various religious coping styles are functional. In view of the strength of connections with other scales, Pargament et al. consider the deferring style to be dysfunctional: "This problem-solving approach was related significantly to a lower sense of personal control, lower self-esteem, less active planful problem-solving skills, less tolerance for individual differences, and a greater sense of control by chance" (1988, 101). As there is no experience with problem-solving scales in the Dutch situation, the conclusion that the deferring style would represent a less adequate way of coping with problems cannot be adopted without question. To acquire some insight in this issue, we used the so-called 'Zelf-Beoordelingsvragenlijst' (ZBV, 'Self-Assessment Questionnaire'), the Dutch adaptation of C.D. Spielberger's 'State-Trait Anxiety Inventory' (Van der Ploeg et al. 1980). The ZBV consists of two scales that allow the measuring of, respectively, state anxiety and trait anxiety. The latter gives a more general impression of the measure of psychological well-being and this makes it more suitable for our purpose (see Pieper et al. 1988). Furthermore, the questionnaire included questions about religious involvement, relig-ious education, and religious role models.

The questionnaire was sent to 500 members (aged between 30 and 65) of local congregations of Protestant churches in the Netherlands. A total of 237 completed questionnaires were returned (a response rate of 47%). 40% of the respondents was male, 60% female (n= 237). Concerning their church membership: 25% belonged to an orthodox Reformed congregation, 40% was Lutheran and 35% belonged to ecumenical Protestant congregations.

A factor analysis (Principal Components Analysis with varimax rotation; missing pairwise; factors= 3; explained variance 53.5% + 10.4% + 7.0% = 70.9%) applied to the translated 'Pargament items' yielded three factors (see Table 1).

Table 1: *Three religious coping styles*

Items	Alma 1998	Pieper & Van Uden 2001
Factor 1: Collaborative	Factor loadings	
When I have a problem, I talk to God about it in my prayers to decide together what it means.	0.79	0.78
When putting my plans into action, I can work together with God.	0.78	0.74
When considering a difficult situation, I put it to God in my prayers in order to think of possible solutions together with Him.	0.78	0.47
When I feel anxious or nervous about a problem, I search in my prayers together with God for a way to relieve my worries.	0.78	Not included
When it comes to deciding how to solve a problem, my faith makes it possible that God and I work together as partners.	0.76	0.69
After solving a problem, I work with God to make sense of it.	0.72	0.72
Factor 2: Self-directing		
When I have some difficulty, I decide what it means by myself without help from God.	0.79	–0.69
When faced with trouble, I deal with my feelings without God's help.	0.77	–0.76
I act to solve my problems without God's help.	0.75	–0.83
When thinking about a difficulty, I try to come up with possible solutions without God's help.	0.71	–0.74
After I've gone through a rough time, I try to make sense of it without relying on God.	0.68	–0.74
When deciding on a solution, I make a choice independent of God's input.	0.66	–0.62

Factor 3: Deferring

Rather than trying to come up with the right solution to a problem myself, I let God decide how to deal with it.	0.76	0.78
I do not think about different solutions to my problems because God provides them for me.	0.76	0.78
When a troublesome issue arises, I leave it up to God to decide what it means for me.	0.74	0.49
When a situation makes me anxious, I wait for God to take those feelings away.	0.74	0.66
In carrying out solutions to my problems, I wait for God to take control and know somehow He'll work it out.	0.72	0.63
I don't spend much time thinking about troubles I've had; God makes sense of them for me.	0.53	Not included

The first factor consists of the six items from the scale that indicates a collaborative style; the second factor contains the six items from the scale that suggests a self-directing style and the third factor contains the six items from the scale that points to a deferring style. The styles appear to correlate, as was also the case in Pargament's study (see Table 2). There is a particularly clear connection between the collaborative and deferring styles: a positive correlation of 0.62. In the case of a high score on the collaborative style scale, respectively the deferring style scale, the score on the self-directing style scale will be lower: negative correlations of –0.76 and –0.52 respectively. The internal consistency of the scales is satisfactory: the reliability analysis yields alpha equal to 0.94 for collaborative, alpha equal to 0.92 for self-directing and alpha equal to 0.85 for deferring. The coping styles seem particularly connected with the respondents' current religious interests (see Table 2).

Especially respondents who stated that they solved their problems together with God, showed a large degree of religious involvement, importance of faith and derived support from faith. Many of them had few doubts about the religious convictions they adopted in childhood. Respondents who indicated that they solved their problems without God's help, scored proportionally low on the variables concerning religious involvement. They were relatively frequently doubtful of the religious convictions that had been handed down to them by their parents and they derived little or no support from their faith (which does not mean that a negative influence was present). It is possible that they had different attitudes towards their faith than is apparent from our coping-questions, but Table 2 shows clearly that this was a group that was less religiously involved and attached less importance to the role faith played in their lives than the other two groups. Respondents with a deferring style showed a similar pattern of answers as that which appeared from the collaborative style items, be it in a less explicit way.

Table 2: *Correlation between the religious coping styles and some variables regarding religiosity (Spearman's rank and partial correlations)*

	Collaborative		Self-directing		Deferring	
	r_s	Partial	r_s	Partial	r_s	Partial
Collaborative						
Self-directing	−0.76					
Deferring	0.62		−0.52			
Religious involvement	0.56	0.35	−0.42	−0.07	0.31	−0.07
Importance of faith	0.62	0.39	−0.48	−0.05	0.41	−0.02
Support from faith	0.65	0.41	−0.54	−0.07	0.40	−0.01
Doubts	−0.35	−0.01	0.41	0.20	−0.31	−0.12

When the independent contribution of the deferring style to the correlations mentioned in the table was calculated (partial correlation), no correlation could be found anymore between the deferring style and the respondents' religious involvement, the importance they attached to their faith and the support they derived from their faith to cope with problems. In keeping with the findings of Pargament *et al.*, faith seemed to be a central, motivating force in the lives of people who scored high on the scale of the collaborative coping style.

As to the Trait Anxiety Scale which was included in the survey: this scale consists of 20 statements with four alternative answers each; therefore the score can range from 20 to 80 points. A person who scores 20 points can be said to have a high degree of psychological well-being; a person who scores 80 points will generally feel anxious and tense. The average score in our sample was 38 points. 32 respondents scored 50 points or over, which showed that their attitude towards life was one of anxiety. There was hardly any connection with the variables as to involvement with church and religiousness and religious education. There was, however, a weak positive correlation with a deferring coping style ($r_s = 0.20$). This indicated that the attitude towards life of respondents who scored high on the deferring coping style scale was, proportionally, more frequently one of anxiety than was the case with respondents with a low score on this scale of coping styles. This was in line with what Pargament *et al.* found in their study carried out among American church members. The correlation, however, was not a strong one and the other coping styles did not show any correlation with the measure for well-being that we had employed.

3. The findings of the study of Pieper & Van Uden (2001)

The shortened and translated version of the 'Three Styles of Religious Coping Scales', as used in Alma's study, was then employed in a study among patients in an Dutch Reformed psychiatric hospital in the Netherlands. All 249 patients treated in 2000 received a questionnaire; 118 questionnaires were returned (a response rate of 47.4%). The age of the participants ranged from 18 to 79 years with a mean of 39 years and a median of 37 years (n= 115). 54% was male, 46% female (n= 116). 97% of the patients was member of a church: 63% Dutch Reformed and 35% Reformed. Apart from the religious coping scales, the questionnaire included questions about the respondents' religious life, about the influence of their religion on their mental problems and about their religious, existential and psychological well-being.

A confirming factor analysis showed that two items of the religious coping scales did not end up in the factors, contrary to what was theoretically expected. These two items were removed from the analysis. This led to a factor solution (Principal Components Analysis with oblique rotation; missing pairwise; factors= 3; explained variance 39.7% + 11.1% + 8.6% = 59.4%) with three factors (see Table 1). From these three factors, scales were constructed with a reliability (alpha) of 0.87, 0.77, 0.81 respectively. On the collaborative scale, scores are highest with 3.15, followed by the self-directing scale (2.60) and the deferring scale (2.56).

From Pargament's study it appeared that the styles were interconnected. This study, too, showed a clear correlation. There was a positive correlation between the deferring and collaborative styles of r= 0.46. The self-directing style contrasted with the other two styles: with the deferring style there was a negative correlation of r= −0.43, but even more so with the collaborative style: a negative correlation of r= −0.63.

The coping styles were connected with the following non-religious and religious characteristics, which were measured in the study by Pieper & Van Uden:

Table 3: *Correlation between the religious coping styles and some non-religious and religious characteristics*
(only significant correlations included)

	Self-directing	Deferring	Collaborative
Self-directing			
Deferring	–0.43		
Collaborative	–0.63	0.46	
Intrinsic	–0.54	0.36	0.48
Positive relation with God	–0.63	0.41	0.62
Private religious activities	–0.28		0.27
Age	–0.35		0.25
Trait anxiety			–0.23

The self-directing style was seen less frequently in intrinsic believers, in patients who had a positive relationship with God, in patients who devoted a great deal of time to private religious activities and in the elderly. The deferring style was seen more frequently in intrinsic believers and in patients who had a positive relationship with God. The collaborative style was seen more frequently in intrinsic believers, in patients who had a positive relationship with God, in patients who devoted a great deal of time to private religious activities and in the elderly. Again it became clear that especially the self-directing and collaborative styles were contrasting styles. The collaborative style (as the only one of the three styles) was connected with the Trait Anxiety Scale: a negative correlation of r= –0.23. This means that a collaborative coping style coincided with lower anxiety levels.

4. Comparison of our findings with those of Pargament *et al.* (1988)

When we compare these findings with Pargament's, we can conclude that the three-factor solution that was found by Pargament *et al.* in 1988, also emerged from the studies carried out by Alma and Pieper & Van Uden, be it that in the latter study two items had to be removed from the analysis. The findings of the studies showed similarities on other points too. As to the correlations among the three factors: they were highest in Alma's study. The study by Pargament *et al.* showed a positive correlation between the collaborative and deferring styles (r= 0.47) and a negative correlation between the collaborative and the self-directing styles (r= –0.61) and the deferring and the self-directing styles (r= –0.37). This pattern is almost identical to that, which emerged from the study carried out by Pieper & Van Uden.

As was the case with the study by Pargament *et al.*, the studies by Alma and Pieper & Van Uden showed that people who used a collaborative style were closest involved in religious issues. At this point, however, it has to be remarked that different measuring instruments have been employed to measure this religious involvement. This also applies to the relation between coping styles and the respondents' competence and well-being. Yet, the findings by Alma, Pieper & Van Uden were in line with the study by Pargament *et al.* who found that a collaborative religious coping style had a more positive effect on the respondents' well-being than a deferring religious coping style. On the whole there was a great deal of similarity as to the findings of the three research projects that had been carried out on different locations and among different populations. Still, we have some criticism.

5. Criticism

When developing the scales for the Alma study, we felt increasingly dissatisfied with the statements that were intended to measure the religious coping styles: careful translation into Dutch revealed their specific American character even more strongly (described by us as an 'unquestioning perception of faith'), and it showed a specific and one-sided view of God (God as the interaction partner who actively intervenes in the individual's life). Another objection to this scale as well as to comparable scales (for example scales measuring religious orientations) was that many statements that assessed a certain style or orientation were in fact synonymous, so that even without a factor analysis they could be predicted to form clusters on the strength of a shared background dimension. The concept validity will suffer from the objections mentioned: one runs the risk that, instead of measuring religious coping styles, one will measure, for example, the degree of resistance to a certain perception of God, or the extent to which respondents identify with the language used in a specific religious tradition. Another risk is that the statements will be completely alien to the respondents, so that they will not be able to choose any of the possible answers on the five-points Likert Scale, or that they will opt for the neutral option, in the middle. This sort of choice is in fact a form of non-response. Furthermore, there is the objection that having to react to a multitude of items, closely resembling each other, will arouse irritation. This appeared to be the case in a pilot questionnaire that was used with a group of researchers at the (Protestant) Vrije Universiteit in Amsterdam, and with fifteen members of a Protestant church. The respondents found it annoying and difficult to react to the religious coping items. In the final survey, we tried to find out what the scales had evoked in the respondents by means of an open, evaluative question at the end of the questionnaire. The reactions collected in this way (that some respondents also had written in the margins next to the statements) underlined that many respondents had had problems especially with the religious coping items.

Although analysing the results of the survey yielded three groups of respondents that corresponded with the three Pargament coping styles, the selection of respondents for interviews in the research conducted by Alma, remained complex. The aim was to select five people from each of the groups for the interviews: respondents with the highest scores on the scale belonging to a particular style. In doing so, however, we had to take into account that there was an overlap between the collaborative and the deferring styles that highly correlate with each other. We opted for either the 'purest' possible collaborative candidates, or the purest deferring ones. It emerged clearly from the interviews that the high correlation between the two styles is a problem because of the poor differentiation between them. Furthermore, the different religious coping styles were not 'pure types': it turned out that, in particular within the group characterised by a deferring style, the respondents experienced and described their relationship with God in completely different ways.

To illustrate this, we briefly summarise here the interview with K., a man in his thirties, who was a member of the Lutheran church. K.'s pattern of answers on the Pargament scales showed a *deferring religious coping style*. However, a certain degree of tension and contradiction between a deferring and a self-directing style could be detected during the interview. That he assumed a deferring attitude could be concluded from what K. said about God's control and guidance, and about acceptance: through an illness and its consequences K. had learned to accept that things are beyond his control and have to run their own course. However, he expressed a self-directing attitude by what he said about being in control himself wherever possible and about Jesus' example ('Simply stand your ground, believe in things. Act. Don't allow yourself to be run over.'). K. thought that healthy, prosperous people like himself could do a lot; they had to assume responsibility for other people who have fewer opportunities. He did not rule out, however, that God's guidance could be at work when he would actually assume this responsibility, for example for his father. K.'s attitude towards life manifested a fighting spirit that, at first sight, could not be reconciled straightaway with a deferring religious coping style. The fact that he did not obtain a higher score on the scale for the collaborative coping style, was presumably due to the God representation that is present in the statements of this Pargament scale. They presume an experience of God's closeness that is alien to K.

The results of the interviews reinforced our conviction that Pargament's grouping fails to do justice to the complexity of religious life. Of course, we realise that over the past years Pargament has tried to optimise his instruments for assessment (for example the RCOPE in: Pargament *et al.* 2000) and he himself has emphasised that "Of course, it would be practically unfeasible to develop scales that reflect methods of coping with all situations by all religious groups" (Pargament *et al.* 2000, 525). Yet, we believe that even the various recently developed scales ignore a crucial dimension. In particular we think that the Pargament scales are focusing too much on a view of an active, personal God and that, therefore, they do not take into account a diffuse relationship with a more impersonal God, that is certainly not uncommon in the secularised Netherlands.

6. In search of a complementary alternative

Apart from translating Pargament's religious coping scales, we have developed a scale that takes into account that people are not always directly focusing on the solution of problems, either with or without God. A receptive attitude might allow them to be open to what they cannot control. This does not refer to the passivity that seems to be characteristic for the deferring style. The point is that people, in actively dealing with a problematic situation, can be open to what might be in store for them. From our point of view, this receptive mode refers to a religious attitude (see Deikman 1982; Schachtel 1959).

We have given this scale the working title 'Fortmann Scale', in view of Fortmann's emphasis on the human being's capabilities of self-actualisation as well as of surrendering as two poles of mental health (Fortmann 1974; see also chapter 1). Pargament *et al.*'s styles for religious coping detach self-actualisation from surrender, which can be found at best in a somewhat 'suspicious' form in the deferring style.

Our scale of religious receptivity consists of three items in which no reference is made to a specific interpretation of a transcendent reality. The items are about trust, finding a deeper meaning, receptivity, and enlightenment. They have been incorporated in a set of twelve items on the analogy of the religious coping scales. The central question of the other nine items is, whether people in troublesome situations assume responsibility and control themselves, or render them to somebody else. Here also, three alternatives are possible: acting independently without help from anybody else (three items), acting together with somebody else (three items), waiting for somebody else to solve the problem (three items).

A factor analysis that we applied to the twelve items, yielded only one factor that allowed adequate interpretation and that consisted of the three Fortmann Scale items. This scale showed a weak positive correlation with both the collaborative style ($r = 0.28$) and the deferring style ($r = 0.23$). Consequently this coping style is closer to the two explicitly God-related religious coping scales than to the self-directing scale.

But so far, unfortunately, the scale has not yielded sufficient information within the framework of our study. This is probably because the three-item version that we used was too short: on the basis of the remarks made in the pilot survey we had considerably shortened the scales discussed here. This was done to counteract irritation triggered by answering the questions on the list that was a long one as such. However, we think that in future research more attention should be paid to this religious-receptive interpretation of coping. Consequently, we intend to further develop our scale of religious receptivity, now consisting of the following three items (see chapter 7 for the final version of our Receptive Coping Scale):

- When I am worried, earlier experiences make me trust that I will be shown a way out.
- After a period of difficulties the deeper significance of my prob-

lems will be revealed to me.
– When I find myself in times of trouble, I have faith in the eventual revelation of their meaning and purpose.

References

Alma, H.A. (1998) *Identiteit door verbondenheid: Een godsdienstpsychologisch onderzoek naar identificatie en christelijk geloof [Identity through Alliance. A Study in the Psychology of Religion on Identification and Christian Faith]*. Kampen: Kok.

Deikman, A.J. (1982) *The Observing Self. Mysticism and Psychotherapy*. Boston: Beacon Press.

Fortmann. H.M.M. (1974) *Als ziende de Onzienlijke. Een cultuurpsychologische studie over de religieuze waarneming en de zogenaamde religieuze projectie (vol.2) [As Seeing Him Who is Invisible. A Cultural Psychological Study of Religious Perception and the So-Called Religious Projection (Vol. 2)]*. Hilversum: Gooi en Sticht.

Oosterwijk, J., Hoenkamp-Bisschops, A., Pieper, J., & Uden, van M.H.F. (1987) *Steun en ontmoeting. Een onderzoek onder bedevaartgangers naar Lourdes [Support and Encounter. A Study of Pilgrims to Lourdes]*. Heerlen: Universiteit voor Theologie en Pastoraat.

Pargament, K.I. (1997) *The Psychology of Religion and Coping. Theory, Research, Practice*. New York: The Guilford Press.

Pargament, K.I., Kennell, J., Hathaway, W., Grevengoed, N., Newman, J., & Jones, W. (1988) Religion and the Problem-Solving Process. Three Styles of Coping. *Journal for the Scientific Study of Religion 27*, 90-104.

Pargament, K.I., Koenig, H.G. & Perez, L.M. (2000) The Many Methods of Religious Coping. Development and Initial Validation of the RCOPE. *Journal of Clinical Psychology 56/4*, 519-543.

Pieper, J.Z.T., Oosterwijk, J.W. & Uden, van M.H.F. (1988) Bedevaart: Steun en ontmoeting. Over de bedevaart naar Lourdes [Pilgrimage: Support and Encounter. On the Pilgrimage to Lourdes]. In: Uden, van M. & Post P. (eds.) *Christelijke bedevaarten. Op weg naar heil en heling [Christian Pilgrimage. On the Road to Salvation and Healing]*. Nijmegen: Dekker & van de Vegt, 159-170.

Pieper, J.Z.T. & Uden, van M.H.F. (2001) *Geestelijke verzorging op De Fontein. Onderzoek onder cliënten van De Fontein naar hun geloof/levensbeschouwing en naar hun behoefte aan geestelijke verzorging [Pastoral Care at De Fontein. Research among Clients of De Fontein regarding their Faith/Worldview and their Need of Pastoral Care]*. Zeist (external report).

Ploeg, van der H.M., Defares, P.B., & Spielberger, C.D. (1980) *Handleiding bij de Zelf-Beoordelingsvragenlijst [Manual of the Self-Assessment Questionnaire]*. Lisse: Swets & Zeitlinger.
Schachtel, E.G. (1959) *Metamorphosis. On the Development of Affect, Perception and Memory*. New York: Basic Books.

CHAPTER 7

"BRIDGE OVER TROUBLED WATER" FURTHER RESULTS REGARDING THE RECEPTIVE COPING SCALE

1. Introduction

Measuring coping has become widespread in the second generation of coping researchers in clinical and social psychology, where it replaced the psychodynamic ego development perspective. This generation emphasises processes rather than structures (personality traits). The processes are treated as transactions between person and environment. In these transactions, cognitions and behaviours are rated more highly than before (Suls *et al.* 1996). Lazarus and Folkman are well-known representatives of this generation. Together with others they developed the Ways of Coping Scale. The scale consists of eight subscales: confrontive coping, distancing, self-control, seeking social support, accepting responsibility, escape-avoidance, planful problem solving and positive reappraisal (Folkman *et al.* 1986). The last subscale contains two religious items: 'found new faith' and 'I prayed'. Carver *et al.* (1989) have extended this scale. Their new scale (COPE) consists of thirteen subscales. The last subscale is called 'turning to religion' and contains four items: 'I seek God's help', 'I put my trust in God', 'I try to find comfort in my religion' and 'I pray more than usual'. In a study of women in treatment for early-stage breast cancer, these items were changed into: 'I've been getting emotional support from the people in my church'; 'I've been going to church or prayer meetings'; 'I've been talking with my priest or minister'; 'I've been trying to find comfort in my religion or spiritual beliefs' (Alferi *et al.* 1999, 347). Parker & Brown (1982) found six dimensions of coping behaviour: recklessness, socialisation, distraction, problem solving, passivity and self-consolation. They used one religious item ('I prayed'). This item was part of the problem-solving dimension. All these scales lack systematic treatment of the place of religion in the coping process.

Psychology of religion has developed measures focusing specifically on religious coping. One measure of religious coping is that of Koenig *et al.* (1992). Their Religious Coping Index (RCI) consists of three items. The first question is open-ended: what enables the subject to cope with stress? A score of 10 was assigned to a religious response (God, prayer etc.). Secondly, subjects are asked to rate the extent to which they use religion to cope on a visual analogue scale ranging from 0 to 10. Finally, the interviewer discusses with subjects how they use religion to cope and asks for specific recent examples. On the basis of the discussion the interviewer rates subjects on a scale of 0 to 10 in respect of their use of religion as a coping behaviour. The three scores are summed. This measure focuses only on the extent to which religion is used in the coping process (quantitative). Specific ways of religious coping (qualitative) are not assessed.

Pargament and his co-researchers followed another road. In 1988 they presented three styles of religious coping in the problem-solving process (Pargament *et al.* 1988). These are: self-directing (the individual is responsible for solving problems), deferring (God is made responsible for problem-solving) and collaborative (both the individual and God are responsible). These styles vary on two key dimensions: God-human being and active-passive. Wong-McDonald suggested an additional coping style: surrender. "Surrender differs from deferring in that it is not a passive waiting for God to solve all problems: rather, it is an active choice to surrender one's will to God's rule" (Wong-McDonald 2000, 149). This style is probably only applicable to the very committed, Bible-oriented believer (it represents the New Testament concept of losing one's life in Christ).

These four religious problem-solving styles measure only a small part of possible religious coping activities. Recently, Pargament *et al.* (2000) developed the RCOPE, a new theoretically based measure that assesses the full range of religious coping methods. "They encompass active, passive, and interactive coping methods. They include problem-focused and emotion-focused approaches. They cover cognitive, behavioural, interpersonal, and spiritual domains" (Pargament *et al.* 2000, 525). The authors discern five main areas, connected to five religious functions: religious coping methods for finding meaning; for gaining control; for gaining comfort and closeness to God; for gaining intimacy with others and closeness to God; and for achieving a transformation of life. Pargament's three religious problem-solving styles are part of the 'gaining control' domain. Two additional styles complete this domain. The first one is pleading for direct intervention. This means seeking control indirectly by pleading to God for a miracle or divine intervention. The second one is active religious surrender, an active handing over of control to God. This means that individuals first try their best, but at a certain point they leave the rest to God. The RCOPE can be divided in two parts: positive and negative religious coping. The RCOPE is a very extensive measure. For that reason, the researchers have also developed an abridged RCOPE (Pargament *et al.* 1998), based on the identification of positive and negative patterns or clusters of religious coping methods.

Earlier we (Alma *et al.* 2003) reported on our attempts to use Pargament's three religious problem solving styles in the Netherlands, the problems we encountered and the alternative scale we tried to develop: the Receptivity Scale. The main problem with Pargament's threefold conceptualisation of religious coping (self-directing, deferring and collaborative) is the underlying view of an active, personal God, which ignores the notion of a more impersonal God that is probably more common in the secularised Netherlands. The Receptivity Scale allows for such an impersonal view of God. Furthermore, the scale takes into account that people do not always focus directly on problem solving, either with or without God. A receptive attitude might allow them to be open to what they cannot control. Confronted with a problematic situation, they may be open to what could be in store for them.

The scale we presented consisted of three items which contained no reference to a specific interpretation of a transcendent reality. The items were about trust, finding deeper meaning, receptivity and enlightenment. The scale yielded some interesting results, but we came to the conclusion that it was too brief and that more attention should be paid to a religiously receptive interpretation of coping in future research. In this chapter we will present a more definitive version of our so-called Receptivity Scale. This version has been administered to two populations in Belgium and two populations in the Netherlands. We will examine the precise meaning of this scale by comparing the respondents' scores on this scale with their scores on other measures of religiosity and other psychological measures. We also compare the scores of theology students with the scores of psychology students. Thus we gain more insight into the validity of the scale.

One of the items in the brief version of the scale was 'When I find myself in times of trouble, I have faith in the eventual revelation of their meaning and purpose'. This reminded us of the Beatles' song "Let it be", in which Mother Mary comes to the singer in times of trouble. In the context of this chapter, Simon & Garfunkel's song "Bridge over troubled water" fits our intentions best. The Receptivity Scale tries to bridge the gap between religious coping with specific reference to a personal God and ways of coping, without a reference to a transcendental reality.

2. The Receptivity Scale

In cooperation with Dirk Hutsebaut and Bart Neyrinck (University of Louvain, Belgium), we first developed a six-item and finally an eight-item version of the Receptivity Scale. (The items in italics were not included in the six-item version):

> People cope with their problems in different ways. Please indicate how often you deal with your problems in the ways described in the following statements. (never/seldom/sometimes/often/always)

1. When I am worried, earlier experiences make me trust that I will be shown a way out.
2. After a period of difficulties the deeper significance of my problems will be revealed to me.
3. When I find myself in times of trouble, I have faith in the eventual revelation of their meaning and purpose.
4. *When I have problems, I trust that a solution will be presented to me.*
5. When I wonder how to solve a problem, I trust that a solution will be shown to me in due course.
6. *In difficult situations I trust that a way out will unfold.*
7. In solving my problems I am sometimes struck by the fact that things just fall into place.
8. In difficult situations I open myself to solutions that arise.

3. Research findings: Hutsebaut and Neyrinck

The Receptivity Scale was administered to various populations. Hutsebaut and Neyrinck used the six-item version in their research in Belgium. The six items were part of a survey that was first conducted with a sample of 225 final year high school and undergraduate students, and then with a second sample of 118 adults, all from the Dutch-speaking part of Belgium. A principal component analysis was carried out on the six items. A scree test pointed to a one-component solution. The six items were used to construct the Receptivity Scale. An estimate of internal consistency (Cronbach's alpha coefficient) was 0.64 (M= 3.31; SD= 0.53). One item, which loaded less than 0.40, was not omitted from the analyses because doing so did not improve internal consistency.

Among the other measures in the survey was a seven-point Likert-type question 'How religious are you?', to measure religiosity, and the Post-critical Belief Scale that captures four approaches to religion: orthodoxy, external critique, relativism and second naïveté. A combination of instruments measured Erikson's concept of basic trust versus basic mistrust; commitment to the transcendent was measured by twelve items from the Spirituality Inventory constructed by Luchtmeijer *et al.* (2001) and finally, the Trait Anxiety part of the State-Trait Anxiety Inventory (STAI) was used. In the adolescent sample, receptivity correlated positively with relativism and second naïveté, two approaches to religion that interpret expressions of religious faith symbolically. It correlated negatively with external critique and not at all with orthodoxy, two approaches to religion that interpret expressions of religious faith literally (see Table 1). In the adult sample, however, receptivity correlated positively with second naïveté and negatively with external critique, whereas it did not correlate with orthodoxy and relativism. In both the adolescent and the adult samples, receptivity correlated positively with religiosity, commitment to the transcendent, and basic trust, and negatively with trait anxiety (see Tables 1 and 2). The correlations were stronger in the adult sample. According to Hutsebaut and Neyrinck, the differences between the adolescent and adult samples are due to the adult sample's stronger involvement in general religiosity.

Table 1: *Correlations between receptivity and the other measures in the survey: adolescent sample*

	Receptivity
Orthodoxy	–0.01
External critique	–0.15*
Relativism	0.34**
Second naïveté	0.29**
Religiosity	0.19*
Commitment to the transcendent	0.37**
Basic trust	0.37**
Anxiety	–0.19*

*n= 225; * p<0.05; ** p<0.01*

Table 2: *Correlations between Receptivity and the other measures in the survey: adult sample*

	Receptivity
Orthodoxy	0.12
External critique	–0.31**
Relativism	–0.07
Second naïveté	0.29**
Religiosity	0.33**
Commitment to the transcendent	0.54**
Basic trust	0.52**
Anxiety	–0.34**

*n= 118; * p<0.05; ** p<0.01*

From these results, Hutsebaut and Neyrinck conclude that religiosity and receptivity do not necessarily go together: it depends on the way an individual approaches religion. In both samples people scoring high on second naïveté – interpreting religion symbolically and including transcendence – can be said to be high in receptivity. It is not surprising that receptivity correlates positively with the symbolic dimension. Both symbolic and receptive thinking can be said to have a certain kind of openness. People scoring high on external critique – interpreting religion literally and excluding transcendence – can be said to be low in receptivity. Literal thinking seems to be the opposite of receptive thinking. Receptivity and basic trust have a strongly positive correlation, but the two concepts are not the same. Receptivity has a stronger positive correlation with commitment to the transcendent than basic trust, whereas basic trust has a stronger negative correlation with anxiety. One might argue that receptivity is an open way of perceiving and thinking about problems, based on basic trust and commitment to the transcendent.

4. Research findings: Alma, Pieper and Van Uden

4.1. Characteristics of the sample

Alma, Pieper and Van Uden used the eight-item version in research in the Netherlands. The sample consisted of 113 subjects: 77 psychology students at the Radboud University Nijmegen and 36 theology students at Leiden University and the Radboud University Nijmegen, respectively. Nineteen percent of the psychology students and 39% of the theology students described themselves as either Protestant or Roman Catholic. Four percent and 28%, respectively, called themselves Christian. Twenty-five percent and 22% respectively adhered to another religion. Eight percent and 11%, respectively referred to themselves as agnostic and 44% and 0%, respectively, as unbelievers (see Table 3).

Table 3: *Religious self-description (%)*

	Psychology	Theology
Protestant / Roman Catholic	19	39
Christian	4	28
Agnostic	8	11
Unbeliever	44	0
Other	25	22

n= 113

As to religious participation, we asked people how often they attended church (see Table 4).

Table 4: *Religious participation: church attendance (%)*

	Psychology	Theology
weekly or often	10	58
only on special occasions	25	19
hardly ever or never	65	22

n= 113

Asked to indicate how religious they were, 55% of the psychology students and 3% of the theology students responded 'not at all'; 14% of the psychology students and 67% of the theology students responded 'very strongly'. Clearly, and as expected, more theology students than psychology students saw themselves as religious.

4.2. Religious coping

In addition to the receptivity items, we presented participants with Pargament's three religious coping style scales. Each of the three subscales consists of six items, which are scored on a five-point Likert Scale (1= 'never', 2= 'seldom', 3= 'sometimes', 4= 'often', 5= 'always'). A Principal Component analysis (with varimax rotation; missing pairwise; mineigen= 1; factor loading >0.40; Explained variance 66.6% + 8.5% = 75.1%; KMO= 0.95) was carried out on the eighteen items and yielded two components (see Table 5).

Table 5: *Two coping factors*

Factor 1: Collaborative versus self-directing

When I have a problem, I talk to God about it in my prayers to decide together what it means.	0.84
When considering a difficult situation, I put it to God in my prayers in order to think of possible solutions together with him.	0.82
When putting my plans into action, I can work together with God.	0.81
When I feel anxious or nervous about a problem, I search in my prayers together with God for a way to relieve my worries.	0.80
When it comes to deciding how to solve a problem, my faith makes it possible that God and I work together as partners.	0.79
After solving a problem, I work with God to make sense of it.	0.72
When thinking about a difficulty, I try to come up with possible solutions without God's help.	–0.84
I act to solve my problems without God's help.	–0.82
When I have difficulty, I decide what it means by myself without help from God.	–0.82
When faced with trouble, I deal with my feelings without God's help.	–0.82
When deciding on a solution, I make a choice independent of God's input.	–0.77
After I've gone through a rough time, I try to make sense of it without relying on God.	–0.76

Factor 2: Deferring

Rather than trying to come up with the right solution to a problem myself, I let God decide how to deal with it.	0.86
I do not think about different solutions to my problems because God provides them for me.	0.82
When a situation makes me anxious, I wait for God to take those feelings away.	0.79
In carrying out solutions to my problems, I wait for God to take control and know somehow he'll work it out.	0.74
When a troublesome issue arises, I leave it up to God to decide what it means for me.	0.72
I don't spend much time thinking about troubles I've had; God makes sense of them for me.	0.58

A forced three-factor solution didn't yield an interpretable result. In the two-factor solution presented here, the collaborative and the self-directing styles are opposite poles of the same factor, with collaborative loading positively, self-directing loading negatively. It is a coping style in which individuals take responsibility themselves or are collaborating with God. Yet, we used the three scales theoretically assumed by Pargament. The estimates of internal consistency (Cronbach's alpha coefficient) are high: 0.96 (collaborative), 0.94 (self-directing) and 0.90 (deferring), respectively. From Pargament's studies, the styles appeared to be interconnected. Our study, too, showed a clear correlation. There was a positive correlation of r= 0.76 between the deferring and collaborative styles. In both styles, God plays an important role. The self-directing style contrasted with the other two styles: with the deferring style (r= –0.70), but even more so with the collaborative style (r= –0.88).

A Principal Component analysis (with varimax rotation; missing pairwise; mineigen= 1; factor loading >0.40) was carried out on the eight receptivity items, again yielding two components (explained variance 42.1% + 18.1% = 60.2%; KMO= 0.77) (see Table 6).

An estimate of internal consistency (Cronbach's alpha coefficient) was 0.78 for factor 1 and 0.70 for factor 2. The items of the first factor refer to an active agent that is present and reveals, presents and shows something. The formulation makes it possible to imagine this agent as a more or less personal God. The items of the second factor seem to refer to opening oneself to fate, or the laws of the cosmos. The agent is absent and something reveals itself.

Table 6: *Two receptivity factors*

Factor 1: Something is revealed by an agent

When I find myself in times of trouble, I have faith in the eventual revelation of their meaning and purpose.	0.80
After a period of difficulties, the deeper significance of my problems is revealed to me.	0.78
When I have problems, I trust that a solution will be presented to me.	0.67
When I wonder how to solve a problem, I trust that a solution will be shown to me in due course.	0.67
When I am worried, earlier experiences make me trust that I will be shown a way out.	0.51

Factor 2: Something reveals itself

In difficult situations I trust that a way out will unfold.	0.81
In solving my problems I am sometimes struck by the fact that things just fall into place.	0.74
In difficult situations I open myself to solutions that arise.	0.72

4.3. Validity

We performed three analysis to gain more insight into the precise meaning of the two receptivity factors. First we correlated the two factors with Pargament's three religious coping styles. The correlations are in line with our interpretation of the two factors and add to our understanding of the receptivity subscales (see Table 7).

Table 7: *Correlations between receptivity and the other religious coping styles*

	Deferring	Collaborative	Self-directing
Receptive-agent	0.44**	0.47**	−0.51**
Receptive-no agent	0.18	0.18	−0.18
Receptive-total	0.41**	0.43**	−0.46**

*n= 113; * p<0.05; ** p<0.01*

We see that receptive-agent is associated with the other religious coping styles (deferring and collaborative), in which a personal God is addressed, and receptive-no agent is not.

Secondly, to gain more information about the precise meaning of the two receptivity scales we correlated them with four other measures: religiosity, psychological well-being, basic trust and commitment to the transcendent.

As in the research of Hutsebaut and Neyrinck, we measured the degree of religiosity with a seven-point Likert-type question, 'How religious are you?'

Psychological well-being was measured on a psychological scale, the ZBV. The ZBV is a self-examination questionnaire that is used to determine the degree of anxiety felt. This questionnaire is the Dutch version of Spielberger's State-Trait Anxiety Inventory (STAI) (Van der Ploeg *et al.* 1980). The ZBV consists of two separate questionnaires which measure two distinct concepts of anxiety, state anxiety and trait anxiety. As we were interested in long-term rather than short-term effects we opted for the Trait Anxiety Scale. This scale consists of twenty statements like 'I feel fine' and 'I feel nervous and agitated'. Ten statements are symptomatically positive and ten are symptomatically negative in their formulation. The response alternatives are: 'hardly ever', 'sometimes', 'often' and 'nearly always'. One can score 1, 2, 3, or 4 points per item. A principal component analysis was carried out on the items. A scree test pointed to a one-component solution. This two-tailed factor could be interpreted as anxiety versus good feeling. Two items, loading less than 0.40, were removed from the analysis ('I lack self-confidence' and 'I am a calm person'). Eighteen items were then used to compute the Anxiety Scale. The scores on the positively formulated items were reversed. The scale was internally consistent (Cronbach's alpha coefficient = 0.88). The scores can range from 18 to 72. The mean score was 34.4 (SD: 7.10).

Erikson's concept of basic trust versus basic mistrust was measured with a combination of instruments. The participants completed a total of thirty items. All items were scored on a five-point Likert-type Scale (1= 'never'; 2= 'seldom'; 3= 'sometimes'; 4= 'often'; 5= 'always'). A principal component analysis was carried out on these items. A scree test plot pointed to a one-component solution. Twelve items loaded less than 0.40 on this component and were removed from the analysis. The remaining 18 items were used to construct the Basic Trust Scale, in which scores of basic mistrust items were reversed. Cronbach's alpha coefficient was 0.87; mean was 66, on item-level 3.67 (i.e. close to 'often').

Commitment to the transcendent was measured by twelve items from the Spirituality Inventory constructed by Luchtmeijer *et al.* (2001). All items were scored on a five-point Likert-type Scale (1=

'never'; 2= 'seldom'; 3= 'sometimes'; 4= 'often'; 5= 'always'). A principal component analysis was carried out on these items. A scree test plot pointed to a one-component solution. One item ('I believe there is a transcendent dimension') only loaded 0.17 on this factor. The remaining eleven items loaded at least 0.40. These eleven items were used to construct the 'commitment to the transcendent' scale. Cronbach's alpha coefficient was 0.95; mean was 32.20, on item-level 2.93 (= 'sometimes').

When we relate these scales to the religious coping scales, we get the following results that underline the discriminatory validity of our scales (see Table 8).

Table 8: *Correlations between religious coping styles and religiosity, anxiety, basic trust and commitment to the transcendent*

	Religiosity	Anxiety	Basic Trust	Transcendent
Receptive-total	0.32**	−0.24*	0.44**	0.51**
Receptive-agent	0.39**	−0.14	0.30**	0.54**
Receptive-no agent	0.05	−0.35**	0.55**	0.25*
Deferring	0.54**	−0.07	0.08	0.56**
Collaborative	0.66**	−0.08	0.11	0.70**
Self-directing	−0.67**	0.07	−0.10	−0.65**

*n= 113; * p<0.05; ** p<0.01*

Receptive-no agent is most clearly negatively related to anxiety and positively to basic trust. It is not related to religiosity and less clearly than receptive-agent to transcendence. Receptive-agent is most clearly related to transcendence and to religiosity, but is also related to basic trust. There is no relation with anxiety. The pattern of the deferring and collaborative relationships with the other variables is the same. The correlations with self-directing are in the opposite direction. This is in line with the correlations between these religious problem-solving styles.

A third and final way to gain more insight into the meaning of the receptivity scales is a comparison between the scores of the theology and psychology students (known group validity). These differences indicate that the former are more inclined to cope with problems in a deferring (mean scores 1.82 vs. 1.34) (F= 16,161; sig.: 0.000; eta^2= 0.13; n= 113), collaborative (mean scores 2.58 vs. 1.61) (F= 22.916; sig.: 0.000; eta^2= 0.17; n= 113) and receptive-agent (mean scores 3.54 vs. 3.20) (F= 6.435; sig.: 0.013; eta^2= 0.06; n= 113) manner. Psychology students are more inclined to cope with problems in a self-directing way (theology 3.35 versus psychology 4.19) (F= 16.681; sig.: 0.000; eta^2= 0.13; n= 113). The scores on receptive-no agent do not differ significantly (mean scores theology students versus psychology students: 3.83 vs. 3.84). Again it is evident that the receptive-agent scale (favoured by theology students) is more associated with religiosity than the receptive-no agent scale. It should also be noted that the psychology students' most commonly used ways of coping are self-directive and receptive-no agent (a largely nonreligious coping pattern). Theology students typically cope in a receptive-no agent and receptive-agent style. The latter is a more religious coping style, but direct reference to a personal God (deferring and collaborative) is not popular.

5. Conclusions

In the introduction we said that the Receptivity Scale tries to bridge the gap between religious coping with reference to a personal God, as measured by Pargament's religious coping style scales, and ways of coping without a reference to a transcendent reality. The items we developed seem to serve this purpose well: in research both in Flanders and in the Netherlands the scale related positively to commitment to the transcendent. The research by Hutsebaut and Neyrinck pointed out that receptivity relates positively to approaches to religion in which the symbolic dimension plays an important part: both symbolic and receptive thinking seems to demand a certain kind of openness in imagining the transcendent. In the research of Alma, Pieper and Van Uden, in which the longer, eight-item version of the Receptivity Scale was used, it was found that this scale consisted of two subscales: one referring indirectly to an *agent* who helps in coping with problems, and another referring to an attitude of trust without feeling helped by an agent. Receptive-agent relates positively to religiosity and to the deferring and collaborative coping styles, in which the person feels helped by God. It relates negatively to the self-directing scale, which can hardly be called a *religious* coping scale. Receptive-no agent, however, does not relate significantly to any of the concepts mentioned. It relates positively to basic trust and to commitment to the transcendent. We can conclude that this coping style is less clearly religious in a traditional sense of belief in God than receptive-agent, but it still differs from basic trust in its positive relationship with a conception of transcendence. From this we conclude that the attitudes of basic trust and trust in a personal God entail different degrees of relating to the transcendent in times of trouble. Receptive-agent comes closer to belief in God, receptive-no agent comes closer to, but is not the same as, basic trust in general. In order to get a clearer view on receptivity, we will conduct further research into these two pillars of our bridge over troubled water.

References

Alferi, S.M., Culver, J.L., Carver, C.S., Arena, P.L. & Antoni, M.H. (1999) Religiosity, Religious Coping, and Distress. A Prospective Study of Catholic and Evangelical Hispanic Women in Treatment for Early-Stage Breast Cancer. *Journal of Health Psychology 4*, 343-356.

Alma, H.A., Pieper, J.Z.T. & Uden, van M.H.F. (2003) When I Find Myself in Times of Trouble: Pargament's Religious Coping Scales in the Netherlands. *Archive for the Psychology of Religion 24*, 64-74.

Carver, C.S., Scheier, M.F. & Weintraub, J.K. (1989) Assessing Coping Strategies. A Theoretically Based Approach. *Journal of Personality and Social Psychology 56*, 267-283.

Folkman, S., Lazarus, R.S., Dunkel-Schetter, C., Delongis, A. & Gruen, R.J. (1986) Dynamics of a Stressful Encounter. Cognitive Appraisal, Coping, and Encounter Outcomes. *Journal of Personality and Social Psychology 50/5*, 992-1003.

Koenig, H.G., Cohen, H.J., Blazer, D.G., Pieper, C., Meador, K.G., Shelp, F., Goli, V. & DiPasquale, B. (1992) Religious Coping and Depression Among Elderly, Hospitalized Medically Ill Men. *American Journal of Psychiatry 149*, 1693-1700.

Luchtmeijer, G., Verbiest, K. & Wouters, I. (2001) *Spiritualiteit, een bepaling van het concept. Een zoektocht naar eenheid in de veelheid [Spirituality, a Conceptualisation. A Quest for Unity within Diversity].* Unpublished manuscript, University of Louvain.

Pargament, K.I., Kennell, J., Hathaway, W., Grevengoed, N., Newman, J. & Jones, W. (1988) Religion and the Problem-Solving Process. Three Styles of Coping. *Journal for the Scientific Study of Religion 27*, 90-104.

Pargament, K.I., Koenig, H.G. & Perez, L.M. (2000) The Many Methods of Religious Coping. Development and Initial Validation of the RCOPE. *Journal of Clinical Psychology 56/4*, 519-543.

Pargament, K.I., Smith, B.W., Koenig, H.G. & Perez, L.M. (1998) Patterns of Positive and Negative Religious Coping with Major Life Stressors. *Journal for the Scientific Study of Religion 37*, 710-724.

Parker, G.B. & Brown, L.B. (1982) Coping Behaviors that Mediate between Life Events and Depression. *Archives of General Psychiatry 39*, 1386-1391.

Ploeg, van der H.M., Defares, P.B. & Spielberger, C.D. (1980) *Handleiding bij de Zelf-Beoordelingsvragenlijst [Manual of the Self-Assessment Questionnaire]*. Lisse: Swets & Zeitlinger.

Suls, J., David, J.P. & Harvey J.H. (1996) Personality and Coping. Three Generations of Research. *Journal of Personality 64/4*, 711-735.

Wong-McDonald, A. (2000) Surrender to God. An Additional Coping Style. *Journal of Psychology and Theology 28*, 149-162.

CHAPTER 8

CLINICAL PSYCHOLOGY OF RELIGION
A TRAINING MODEL

In this chapter we will present part of a course in "Clinical Psychology of Religion", that has been developed in the Netherlands with the aim of introducing mental health professionals to the field of the clinical psychology of religion. Clinical psychology of religion aims at applying insights from general psychology of religion to the field of clinical psychology. Clinical psychology of religion can be defined as that part of the psychology of religion that deals with the relation between religion, worldview and mental health. Like the clinical psychologist, the clinical psychologist of religion deals with psychological assessment and psychotherapy, but concentrates on the role religion or worldview play in mental health problems. In recent research (see chapter 3) we have found that there is a great need among psychotherapists to become better equipped in this area.

1. Introduction

In a review of ten years (1984-1994) of research regarding religion and psychotherapy, Worthington *et al.* (1996) indicate that, since 1986, the interest in religion and counselling has been booming. In the last few years in the Netherlands the interest in the relation between meaning giving, worldview and religion on the one hand, and social and mental health care on the other, is growing too.

What does this mean for the practice of mental health care in the Netherlands? As we said in chapter 2 there is agreement that religion and worldview could and should have a prominent place in many psychotherapeutic interventions. The physical, emotional, behavioural and social problems that clients bring in, are often related to their systems of meaning and to their religious attitudes. At the same time, psychotherapists are being accused of neglecting this dimension. Some authors, in particular those who are close to the Protestant tradition, are specifically concerned about their clients' religious values (Schilder 1991; Van der Wal 1991). In the latter group there are also authors who argue that clergy should be working in the institutions for regional community mental health care (the so-called Riaggs), and there are even authors who advocate founding new regional community mental health care institutions based on Christian principles, of which the Gliagg is an example. Representatives of the Riagg however disagree. They state that even in the very religious regions in the Netherlands there are enough Riagg therapists with sufficient expertise in clients' religious backgrounds.

How do the Riagg and the Gliagg therapists themselves evaluate the place of religion/worldview in their own lives and practices?

Let us summarise the main conclusions from our research (Pieper & Van Uden 1998a; 1998b; Schuurman et al. 1999; Van Uden & Pieper 2000) regarding these issues (see also chapters 2 and 3 in this volume).

1. With respect to the religious backgrounds of the Riagg therapists, the following conclusion was drawn. Compared with Dutch citizens in general, therapists believed less in God and had a lower rate of weekly church attendance. The response rate of 49% was also an indication that the research topic was not particularly interesting to the therapists of these non-religious Riaggs. At the Gliagg the response rate was 76%. For the Gliagg therapists, faith was a fundamental value. They all believed in God and attended church at least once a week.

2. With respect to the relation between religion/worldview and mental problems, the following conclusions were drawn. Earlier research (Pieper & Van Uden 1996; Van Uden & Pieper 1996; 1998) had shown that 40% of clients reported a relationship between these two variables. Riagg therapists reported that they saw such a relationship in only 18% of their clients. The Gliagg therapists reported this relationship in 67% of their clients. With regard to the nature of the relationship, we concluded that clients themselves pointed more to the positive influence of religion/worldview than did the Riagg therapists. Of the Riagg therapists who saw a relation, half saw a positive one, half saw a negative one. The Gliagg therapists, on the other hand, pointed more to the positive influence of faith.

3. With respect to the actual treatment of religious/worldview aspects of mental problems, most Riagg therapists claimed to examine

these aspects. But at the same time, half of them were not confident about their skills in treating these aspects, and this led to a need for more training (46%). Specific religious techniques were hardly used.

All Gliagg therapists said they dealt with the religious/worldview aspects of mental problems and used several religious techniques. 41% of them prayed privately for their clients. 80% felt confident about their skills in dealing with religious problems. Yet, 57% would like to receive more training in this area.

4. Contacts between Riagg therapists and clergy were rather few. Referral occurred in only about 1% of cases. In the Gliagg, the contacts were substantial. The Gliagg therapists knew how to contact clergy and had confidence in their competence.

Most relevant in the present context are the facts that 46% of the Riagg therapists stated that they would like to receive more training in the area of religion and worldview, and that even 57% of the Gliagg therapists stated the same.

2. The course

Here we will present part of a course in "Clinical Psychology of Religion", that has been developed in the Netherlands with the aim of introducing mental health professionals to the field of the clinical psychology of religion.

The aim is to help these professionals to acquire more specific knowledge and skills regarding the ways in which mental health problems are related to religion or worldview in general. A related aim of the course is to prepare them for activities in these areas where clients turn to professionals for help in understanding and solving psychological problems that are related to meaning, religion and worldview. More specifically, the course aims at three objectives:

1. The mental health worker should acquire specific knowledge with respect to theories and concepts that help to understand the search for meaning in life as a cognitive appraisal process, how religion and other sociocultural systems are involved in this process, and how the construction of meaning is related to self-esteem, subjective well-being, and psychopathology.

2. The mental health worker should acquire theoretical competence in relating clinical psychological theories and concepts to the field of

religion, and theories and concepts of the psychology of religion to behavioural phenomena in the domain of psychopathology and mental health.

3. The mental health worker should acquire basic practical skills for working in a mental health care agency, as a professional focussed on mental health problems that obviously or presumably are related to religion.

The content of the course deals with the clinical psychology of religion. Just like the clinical psychologist, the clinical psychologist of religion has to deal with psychological assessment and psychotherapy. He is focussed, however, on the role of religion or worldview in mental health problems. The clinical psychology of religion applies the knowledge of the general psychology of religion to the field of the clinical psychologist. Psychological processes like projection, rationalisation, and other defence mechanisms serving to overcome anxiety, have always been expressed in various forms of religious behaviour (dogmatism, intolerance, taboos, utopias, and so on). Anxiety is one of the roots of religiosity. Another root lies in the basic human experience of the search for meaning. In spite of the destabilisation of overarching frameworks of meaning and the marginalisation of church and religion, these psychological structures remain active and become manifest in more secularised ways.

To summarise, the clinical psychology of religion is involved (a) in pathology that is expressed in religious phenomena, and (b) in the search for meaning. When people feel disintegrated as a consequence of serious illness or other traumatic events, a reappraisal of the meaning of life is necessary for the recovery to psychological well-being. The clinical psychology of religion can be described as that part of the psychology of religion that is specifically involved in the relation between religion, worldview, and mental health.

We will now introduce the principles of the specific method, the so-called Problem Oriented Education procedure, that we have used to unfold the field of the clinical psychology of religion.

3. Principles and characteristics of Problem Oriented Education

Most readers will be familiar with situations in which someone asks them about something they should know (ready knowledge, previously learned material). They know that they know it. They can visualise the pages in the book or the words on the blackboard in front of them. Yet the knowledge is not accessible, they cannot give an answer.

In some professions there is not enough time to immediately look up the answers in the literature. Nor is it always easy to reason appropriately about problems. Which approach is best? In practice, a problem is often more complex than one specific discipline's approach would lead one to expect.

Academic education developed Problem Oriented Education as a solution to this sort of situations. Since its introduction in 1969 at McMaster University in Hamilton, Canada, many universities and institutes of higher education have implemented Problem Oriented Education. In the Netherlands, for example, courses in the curriculum at Maastricht University have been given a 'problem oriented' form.

3.1. Problem Oriented Education: Starting points

In Problem Oriented Education, acquiring and applying specialised knowledge go hand in hand. This makes the students' specialised knowledge accessible and usable.

This goal is achieved by using assignments as a teaching tool. Assignments consist of carefully selected problem situations that describe phenomena or events that one may be confronted with in one's professional life.

Assignments encourage students to ask themselves what they would do in such a situation, or what they would think about it. Almost automatically they will ransack their thoughts for similar situations or events that they may have experienced and for concepts they can use to analyse the event or phenomenon. In other words, they will activate their prior knowledge. They will also direct their own learning processes. They will link the professional knowledge they are acquiring to their present knowledge and interests.

Working out assignments and learning with the help of the described phenomena or events (problem situations) is not something students do on their own. They discuss the assignment in a study group, observing a procedure known as the 'zevensprong' ('jumping in seven steps', named after an old folk dance). They articulate the problem together, analyse it using what they, as a group, already know, and formulate questions for further study. Using these questions, each group member studies the literature individually trying to arrive at a solution or at a more precise formulation of the problem. The results are discussed in the study group chaired by one of the group members. Together they deal with the problem and draw conclusions. A tutor facilitates the study group. This is the lecturer's role. The tutor guides the discussion and the learning process only when necessary. While working on the assignment, students get direct feedback regarding their progress, from their fellow group members as well as their tutor.

In short, they work in a study group and in independent study activities on assignments, in which a problem is formulated that is to serve as a model for a whole spectrum of equivalent problems in their professional lives. They immediately apply what they learn to the problem.

3.2. Method

In Problem Oriented Education students get several assignments. These are intended to develop skills and to apply them immediately. Each assignment (via a text, a film or a video) describes or refers to a situation they could meet in their professional lives.

It is not immediately clear what the problem is, let alone what the solution is, and at least there is no immediately obvious 'professional' solution that does justice to the complexity of the problem.

The students analyse the problem and suggest possible solutions. They are expected to display an active and independent study attitude in analysing, together with other group members, the problem, and to develop a usable expertise in 'handling' such problems.

One of the tools for learning how to approach problems systematically and scientifically is the 'zevensprong'. It is a step by step way of solving problems that arise, or of better defining them.

3.3. The 'Zevensprong'

Before joining the study group, the students study at home the assignment that will be discussed at the meeting. They examine it guided by the following questions, making notes that they can use during the study group meeting:

- What are the essential points described or raised in the problem situation?
- What problem has, in your opinion, been formulated, or would have to be formulated, in this assignment?
- In regard to which important or difficult concepts have you been unable to find a meaning?

Steps 1 to 5 (see below) take place in the study group as a preparation for step 6, independent study, and step 7, the return to the ('improved' and more professional) statement of the problem.

Step 1 – Confrontation with the assignment
tasks: A first exploration. Description of difficult concepts. Extracting the important points from the assignment. Arriving, as a group, at a first provisional working definition.

Step 2 – Formulating the problem
tasks: A concise formulation of the problem that, in the group's view, is present in this assignment. This formulation should include all the important points (see step 1) present in the assignment.

Articulation of the problem as a question to be investigated, not to be judged.

Step 3 – Analysing the problem
tasks: Brainstorming about the elements that could play a role in analysing the problem. All group members participate, applying their previously acquired knowledge.

Step 4 – Stock-taking
tasks: Structuring (stock-taking and ordering) of the factors that play a role in the problem (brainstorming phase) and that offer material for a possible explanation or illumination of the problem.

Step 5 – Formulating learning goals
tasks: Drafting study questions to use in dealing with the problem. Study questions refer to concepts the working definitions of which have been agreed upon, and to relations between factors that may explain or illuminate the problem.

Step 6 – Independent study

Guided by the problem formulation and the study questions, students select and study relevant literature. They take notes so that

(a) their study questions are answered;

(b) using the literature studied and their notes, they can process the problem as formulated.

In this way they prepare for the following meeting of the study group where the assignment will be discussed further.

tasks: Targeted examination of the literature using the study questions; preparation for processing the problem in the study group.

Step 7 – Returning to the problem

This step takes place during the next study group meeting.

tasks: Processing of the problem using the results of independent study (step 6). This means confronting the results of their independent study with the (provisional) formulation of the problem (step 2) and with the interpretations / study results of the other group members.

3.4. The study group

It is usual for one meeting to precede the assignment and another one to follow it. Each discussion of each assignment, the one preceding it as well as the one following it, is chaired by one of the group members, who take turns in fulfilling this function.

Before each discussion, a minutes secretary is appointed to write the important points on a blackboard.

In principle, neither the chairperson nor the minutes secretary actively contribute to the content of the discussion. The tutor, normally a lecturer, is watching over, guiding and advancing the content of the discussions. This duty does not take the form of actively contributing to the content.

4. Clinical psychology of religion in eight assignments

In our course we unfold the field of clinical psychology of religion by means of eight successive learning assignments. In the Problem Oriented Education procedure, the learning assignments will be completed in a series of nine meetings. In the first three assignments ('religion and mental health', 'mystical experience and psychopathology' and 'religion and depression'), the focus is on the relation between religion and mental health/illness. The first on tackles it in a general way, then a religious phenomenon (mystical experience) is approached from the perspective of mental illness, and after that a psychological disorder (depression) is related to specific religious belief structures. In the fourth assignment (projection), the fundamental question is discussed, whether or not religiosity can be reduced to psychological processes. Is religion merely projection or is it more than that? In the fifth assignment, we deal with religious imagination. In the sixth, we discuss religion as a coping device. The last two assignments ('religious countertransference' and 'psychotherapy and pastoral care') are practice-oriented and focus on the treatment of religious problems in mental health care.

In sum, we have the following topics: 1. Religion and mental health; 2. Mystical experience and psychopathology; 3. Religion and depression; 4. Projection; 5. Religious imagination; 6. Religion as a coping device; 7. Religious countertransference; 8. Psychotherapy and pastoral care.

4.1. One of the assignments by way of illustration

To conclude, we will illustrate the procedure by presenting one of the assignments. We have selected the one dealing with countertransference. The study group is confronted with the following situation:

Assignment 7: Religious Countertransference
Instruction: Steps 1-5 of the "zevensprong"
Material:
A 42 year old female who is experiencing marital difficulties comes for counselling at a counselling centre. The client belongs to a small Baptist congregation in a semi rural area; the counsellor, who is also female, is divorced and at present she is

Episcopalian (formerly she was a member of a fundamentalist Bible Christian Church). Initially, the client has asked for some coping mechanisms and for ideas on how to communicate better with her husband. After a number of sessions, the severity and complexity of the problem has come more to the surface. Consequently, the picture of the presenting complaint, which had been vague and had each time been introduced with a strong statement about the importance of the sacredness of marital commitment, has become clearer.

In addition, the client has begun to describe some changes in the family that are sources of additional pressure. Married at 18, she had wanted to move out of her parents' home that was quite strict and to start a family of her own with a man whom she perceived as 'strong'. Initially the marriage had seemed quite calm. When asked about this she noted that her traditional role of wife and mother had made her feel fulfilled, and apart from her husband's occasional flare-ups, the match had seemed 'satisfactory'. Most of her efforts had been centred on her family and activities in the church.

In her late 30s, several significant changes had taken place. The children, by now grown-ups, had left home.

Client (Cl): "I was so upset I didn't know what to do, so I went to the minister. I told him all about it and he seemed to be sympathetic."

Counsellor (Co): "Seemed to be?"

Cl: "Well he was very sorry for me but said that it was God's will that I had this tribulation in my life and that I should pray very hard."

Co: "That didn't seem to be exactly what you hoped to hear from him, did you?" (Counsellor is feeling furious at this point and would like to both point out – from her viewpoint – the terrible theology and lack of empathy in the minister's statement; her "gut feeling" is to say, "He's a jerk; why didn't you tell the chauvinist pig to go to hell!")

Cl: "Well no. I guess I expected him to tell me how to make the situation better somehow. But that's not the end of it. I then said to him that I didn't know how long I could take the abuse and that maybe I would have to separate from my husband. At that point he really got wild. He said that women were subject to their husbands and pulled out the Bible to show me where it was written. He said it was evil for me to even think that and I was avoiding my responsibilities as a Christian woman."

Co: (The counsellor is now furious inside.) "How did you feel when he responded this way?"

Cl: "Well, I became frightened. I was also sad. I want to be a good wife. But it's so hard. I felt sort of guilty asking about the separation; I knew I was wrong, but it has been so hard." (Pause)

Co: (Counsellor feels like rescuing client.) "So, you have had it so hard that you even thought of leaving your husband and you went to the minister for some support and instead he yelled at you."

Cl: "Yea. I hoped he would help me out of this mess. Now I feel like it's worse..." (Client looks directly at counsellor.) "Do you think I should leave my husband... I mean is it ok? I know you're not from my church but do you think it's a sin?"

Co: (Counsellor feels like saying, "Of course it's no sin; the sooner you are away from that bastard and your small-minded minister, the better off you'll be!").

[*From:* Wicks, R.J. (1985) My Values, your Values: my Defences, your Defences. Counter-transference with Clients of Different Religious Denominations. *Journal of Pastoral Counselling 20,* 47-52.]

Independent Study: Step 6 of the "zevensprong"
Returning to the Problem: Step 7 of the "zevensprong"
Literature relevant to this assignment:

J.H.N. Kerssemakers (1989) Tegenoverdracht bij religieuze problematiek [Countertransference with respect to religious problems]. In: J.H.N. Kerssemakers. *Psychotherapeuten en religie. Een verkennend onderzoek naar tegenoverdracht bij religieuze problematiek [Psychotherapists and Religion. An Exploratory Study of Countertransference with Respect to Religious Problems].* Nijmegen: Katholiek Studiecentrum, 31-38.

Uleyn, A.J.R. (1986) Zingevingsvragen en overdrachtsproblemen in de psychotherapie [Questions about Meaning and Transference Problems in Psychotherapy]. In: Kuilman, M. & Uleyn, A.J.R. *Hulpverlener en zingevingsvragen [The Helping Professions and Questions about Meaning].* Baarn: Ambo, 35-67.

Recommended literature:

Pruyser, P.W. (1971) Assessment of the Patients' Religious Attitudes in the Psychiatric Case Study. *Bulletin of the Menninger Clinic 35,* 272-291.

Shafranske, E.P. & Newton Malony H. (1990) Clinical Psychologists'
Religious and Spiritual Orientations and their Practice of Psychotherapy. *Psychotherapy 27*, 72-78.

Wicks, R.J. (1985) My Values, your Values: my Defences, your Defences. Countertransference with clients of Different Religious
Denominations. *Journal of Pastoral Counselling 20*, 47-52.

Yalom, I.D. (1992) *When Nietzsche Wept.* New York: Basic Books.

5. Conclusion

We hope that we have been able to make clear that this teaching procedure is able to stimulate study in the area of the clinical psychology
of religion in a fresh way, in particular for workers in the field of mental health care, who tend to be rather distant from religious issues. Research as to the actual effects of the course has yet to be done, but we
are quite optimistic. In our experience, this procedure and this course
have been able to (re-?)create an intrinsic interest in religious issues
among these highly secularised professionals. Apart from this, another
effect has been that several of the groups of participants have become
quite close and have started to function as peer supervision groups
regarding religious and worldview topics in psychotherapy.

References

Pieper, J.Z.T. & Uden, van M.H.F. (1996) Religion in Mental Healthcare.
Patients' views. In: Verhagen, P.J. & Glas, G. (eds.) *Psyche and Faith.
Beyond Professionalism.* Zoetermeer: Boekencentrum, 69-83.

Pieper, J.Z.T., Uden, van M.H.F. (1998a) Religieuze hulpverlening. Gliagg-
therapeuten over geloof en levensbeschouwing [Religious Treatment.
Gliagg Therapists' Views on Faith and Worldview]. In: Uden van M. &
Pieper, J. (eds.). *Wat baat religie? Godsdienstpsychologen en godsdienstsociologen over het nut van religie [Religion to What Avail? Psychologists and Sociologists of Religion on the Benefits of Religion].* Nijmegen:
KSGV, 47-66.

Pieper, J.Z.T. & Uden, van M.H.F. (1998b) Riagg-therapeuten over geloof en
levensbeschouwing [Riagg Therapists' Views on Faith and Worldview].
In: Janssen, J., Uden, van M, & Ven, van der J. (eds.) *Schering en inslag.
Opstellen over religie in de hedendaagse cultuur [Normal Practice. Essays on Religion in Present-Day Culture].* Nijmegen: KSGV, 52-74.

Schilder, A. (1991) Eigen over- of ongevoeligheden t.a.v. een christelijke levensbeschouwing [Our Own Hypersensitivities or Insensitivities towards a Christian Worldview]. In: Filius, R. & Visch, M. (eds.) *Zin in Welzijn. Over levensbeschouwing en professionaliteit in het welzijnswerk. [Meaning in Well-Being. About Worldview and Professionality in Welfare Work]*. Zwolle: Studiecentrum Welzijnswerk en Levensbeschouwing Windesheim, 41-49.

Schuurman, I., Uden, van M.H.F. & Pieper, J.Z.T. (1999) Meer licht op levensbeschouwing in therapie. Een kwalitatief onderzoek naar levensbeschouwing onder Gliagg- en Riagg-therapeuten [More Light on Worldview in Therapy. A Qualitative Investigation among Gliagg and Riagg Therapists]. *Psyche & geloof 10*, 100-115.

Uden, van M.H.F. & Pieper, J.Z.T. (1996) *Religie in de geestelijke gezondheidszorg [Religion in Mental Health Care]*. Nijmegen: KSGV.

Uden, van M.H.F., Pieper, J.Z.T. (1998) Geloof en levensbeschouwing in de geestelijke gezondheidszorg [Faith and Worldview in Mental Health Care]. In: Glas, G. (eds.). *Psychiatrie en religie. De bijna verloren dimensie [Psychiatry and Religion. The Nearly-Lost Dimension]*. Nijmegen: KSGV, 75-97.

Uden, van M.H.F., Pieper, J.Z.T. (2000) Religion in Mental Health Care. Psychotherapists' Views. *Archiv für Religionspsychologie 23*, 264-277.

Wal, van der J. (1991) *Principes en praxis van gereformeerde hulpverlening [Principles and Practice of Reformed Mental Health Care]*. Lezing op studiemiddag 'Riagg en geloof'. Tiel.

Wicks, R.J. (1985) My Values, your Values: my Defences, your Defences. Countertransference with clients of Different Religious Denominations. *Journal of Pastoral Counselling 20*, 47-52.

Worthington, E.L. Jr., Kurusu, T.A., McCullough, M.E. & Sandage, S.J. (1996) Empirical Research on Religion and Psychotherapeutic Processes and Outcomes. A 10-year Review and Research Prospectus. *Psychological Bulletin 119*, 448-478.

BIBLIOGRAPHY

Alferi, S.M., Culver, J.L., Carver, C.S., Arena, P.L. & Antoni, M.H. (1999) Religiosity, Religious Coping, and Distress. A Prospective Study of Catholic and Evangelical Hispanic Women in Treatment for Early-Stage Breast Cancer. *Journal of Health Psychology 4*, 343-356.

Allport, G.W. (1950) *The Individual and his Religion*. New York: Macmillan.

Allport, G.W. & Ross, J.M. (1967) Personal Religious Orientation and Prejudice. *Journal of Personality and Social Psychology 5*, 432-443.

Alma, H.A. (1998) *Identiteit door verbondenheid. Een godsdienstpsychologisch onderzoek naar identificatie en christelijk geloof [Identity through Alliance. A Study in the Psychology of Religion on Identification and Christian Faith]*. Kampen: Kok.

Alma, H.A., Pieper, J.Z.T. & Uden, van M.H.F. (2003) When I Find Myself in Times of Trouble: Pargament's Religious Coping Scales in the Netherlands. *Archive for the Psychology of Religion 24*, 64-74.

Argyle, M. & Beit-Hallahmi, B. (1975) *The Social Psychology of Religion*. London: Routledge and Kegan Paul.

Augustine (1998) *The Confessions* (Transl. Maria Boulding OSB). New York: Vintage Books (Vintage Spiritual Classics).

Baker, M. & Gorsuch, R. (1982). Trait Anxiety and Intrinsic-Extrinsic Religiousness. *Journal for the Scientific Study of Religion 21*, 119-122.

Bauduin, D. (red.) (1991) *Herzuiling in de GGZ? Meningen en discussie over de relatie tussen levensbeschouwing en geestelijke gezondheidszorg in de jaren negentig ['Re-Pillarisation' in Mental Health Care? Opinions and Debates about the Relationship between Worldview and Mental Health Care in the Nineties]*. Utrecht: NcGv.

Bergin, A.E. (1983) Religiosity and Mental Health. A Critical Re-evaluation and Meta-Analysis. *Professional Psychology: Research and Practice 14*, 170-184.

Bergin, A.E., Jensen, J.P. (1990) Religiosity of Psychotherapists. A National Survey. *Psychotherapy 27*, 3-7.

Bernstein, M. (1978) *Nonnen. Van een mysterieus bestaan achter kloostermuren naar de emancipatie van een oude levensstijl. [Nuns. From a Mysterious Existence behind Convent Walls to the Emancipation of an Old Life Style].* Baarn: In den Toren.

Boisen, A.T. (1952) The General Significance of Mystical Identification in Cases of Mental Disorder. *Psychiatry 15*, 287-296.

Carver, C.S., Scheier, M.F. & Weintraub, J.K. (1989) Assessing Coping Strategies. A Theoretically Based Approach. *Journal of Personality and Social Psychology 56*, 267-283.

Clark, W.H. (1958) *The Psychology of Religion*. New York: Macmillan.

Conway, F. & Siegelman, J. (1979) *Knappen [Snapping]*. Amsterdam/Brussel: Elsevier.

Daaleman, T.P. (1999) Belief and Subjective Well-being in Outpatients. *Journal of Religion and Health 38*, 219-227.

Deikman, A.J. (1982) *The Observing Self. Mysticism and Psychotherapy*. Boston: Beacon Press.

Dekker, G., Hart, de J. & Peters, J. (1997) *GOD in Nederland, 1966-1996. [GOD in the Netherlands 1966-1996]*. Amsterdam/Hilversum: Anthos/RKK/KRO.

Derks, F., Pieper, J. & Uden, van M. (1991). Transformatie en confirmatie. Interviews met bedevaartgangers naar Wittem en Lourdes [Transformation and Confirmation. Interviews with Pilgrims to Wittem and Lourdes]. In: Uden, van M., Pieper, J. & Henau, E. (eds.) *Bij Geloof. Over bedevaarten en andere uitingen van volksreligiositeit [Faith or Superstition? On Pilgrimages and Other Forms of Popular Religion]*. Hilversum: Gooi en Sticht, 105-123.

Derksen H. (1994) *De parel in het zwarte doosje. De rol van het geloof in de psychische problemen van katholieke Limburgse vrouwen [The Pearl in the Black Box. The Role of Faith in the Mental Problems of Roman Catholic Women in Limburg]*. Nijmegen: De Wetenschapswinkel Nijmegen.

Dijkhuis, J.H. & Mooren, J.H.M. (1988) *Psychotherapie en levensbeschouwing [Psychotherapy and Worldview]*. Baarn: Ambo.

Dost, A.J. (1992). Riagg en levensbeschouwing. Een persoonlijke ervaring [Riagg and Worldview: A Personal Experience]. In: Damen, E., Wurff, van der A. & Aberson, J. *Levensbeschouwing en de Riagg. Verleden, heden en toekomst [Worldviews and Riagg. Past, Present and Future]*. Zwolle: Riagg-Zwolle.

Draak, den C. (1990) *Lezing kennismakingsbijeenkomst Riagg-Zwolle – Geestelijke Verzorgers regio Zwolle op 19 februari en 19 maart 1990 [Presentation at Introductory Meeting of Riagg Zwolle and Zwolle Area Chaplains, 19 February and 19 March 1990]*. Zwolle: Hogeschool Windesheim/Riagg-Zwolle.

Draak, den C. & Kleingeld, K. (1991) *Levensbeschouwing in het welzijnswerk. Verslag van een praktijkgericht onderzoek naar de rol van levensbeschouwing bij bestuurs- en direktieleden, uitvoerend werkers en cliënten van twee confessionele instellingen voor welzijnswerk [Worldviews in Welfare Work. Report on a Practice-Oriented Investigation of the Role of Worldviews in Board and Executive Members, Staff and Clients of Two Confessional Welfare Work Agencies]*. Zwolle: Studiecentrum Welzijnswerk en Levensbeschouwing Windesheim.

Easton, A. (1990) *Bejaardenoorden en levensbeschouwing. Deel 1: Begripsbepaling, beleid en thematische uitwerkingen [Homes for the Elderly and Worldview. Vol. 1: Concepts, Policies and Thematic Elaborations]*. Amstelveen: Algemene Vereniging van Instellingen voor Bejaardenzorg.

Fabricatore, A.N., Handal, P.J. & Fenzel, L.M. (2000) Personal Spirituality as a Moderator of the Relationship between Stressors and Subjective Well-Being. *Journal of Psychology & Christianity 19*, 221-228.

Filius, R. & Visch, M. (eds.) (1991) *Zin in welzijn. Over levensbeschouwing en professionaliteit in het welzijnswerk [Meaning in Well-Being. About Worldview and Professionality in Welfare Work]*. Zwolle: Studiecentrum Welzijnswerk en Levensbeschouwing Windesheim.

Fitchett, G., Burton, L.A. & Sivan, A.B. (1997) The Religious Needs and Resources of Psychiatric Inpatients. *The Journal of Nervous and Mental Disease 185*, 320-326.

Folkman, S. & Lazarus, R.S. (1980) An Analysis of Coping in a Middle-aged Community Sample. *Journal of Health and Social Behaviour 21*, 219-239.

Folkman, S., Lazarus, R.S., Dunkel-Schetter, C., Delongis, A. & Gruen, R.J. (1986) Dynamics of a Stressful Encounter. Cognitive Appraisal, Coping, and Encounter Outcomes. *Journal of Personality and Social Psychology 50/5*, 992-1003.

Fortmann, H.M.M. (1974) *Als ziende de Onzienlijke (deel 1 en 2) [As Seeing Him Who is Invisible (Vols. 1 and 2)].* Hilversum: Gooi en Sticht.

Freud, S. (1907) *Zwangshandlungen und Religionsübungen [Obsessive Actions and Religious Practices].* Freud Studienausgabe, 1975, Band 7, 11-21. Frankfurt: Fischer Verlag.

Freud, S. (1927) *Die Zukunft einer Illusion [The Future of an Illusion].* Gesammelte Werke, 1961, Band 14, London.

Galanter, M., Rabkin, R., Rabkin, J. & Deutsch, A. (1979) The Moonies. A Psychological Study of Conversion and Membership in a Contemporary Religious Sect. *American Journal of Psychiatry 136*, 165-169.

Goodman, F.D. (1972) *Speaking in Tongues. A Cross-Cultural Study of Glossolalia.* Chicago: University of Chicago Press.

Groen, de I. & Slockers-Beverwijk, G. (1987) *Religie en psychotherapie. Literatuuronderzoek en een onderzoek op twee Riagg's. Doctoraalscriptie vakgroep klinische psychologie, Rijksuniversiteit Leiden. [Religion and Psychotherapy. Literature Review and an Investigation in Two Riaggs. 'Doctoraal' Dissertation Dept. of Clinical Psychology, State University Leiden].*

Gyselen, M. (1979). Mijn patiënt was meer dan ziek [My Patient was More than Just Ill]. In: Gyselen, M. *et al. Hoe menselijk is mystiek? [How Human is Mysticism?].* Baarn: Ambo.

Harrison, M.O. (2001) The Epidemiology of Religious Coping. A Review of Recent Literature. *International Review of Psychiatry 13*, 86-96.

Hart, van der O. (1984) *Rituelen in psychotherapie. Overgang en bestendiging. [Rituals in Psychotherapy. Transition and Confirmation].* Deventer: Van Loghum Slaterus.

Hart, van der O. *et al.* (1981) *Afscheidsrituelen in psychotherapie [Leavetaking Rituals in Psychotherapy].* Baarn: Ambo.

Hoenkamp, A. (1991) *Varianten van celibaatsbeleving. Een verkennend onderzoek rond ambtscelibaat en geestelijke gezondheid. [Varieties of Celibacy Experience. An Exploratory Investigation of Official Celibacy and Mental Health].* Baarn: Ambo.

Hoge, D.R. (1972) A Validated Intrinsic Religious Motivation Scale. *Journal for the Scientific Study of Religion 11*, 369-376.

James, W. (1902) *The Varieties of Religious Experience. A Study in Human Nature.* New York: Modern Library Press, 1994 (original 1902).

Janssen, J., Hart, de J. & Draak, den C. (1989) Praying Practices. *Journal of Empirical Theology 2*, 28-39.

Jenkins, R.A. & Pargament, K.I. (1995) Religion and Spirituality as Resources for Coping with Cancer. *Journal of Psychosocial Oncology 13*, 51-74.

Kennedy, E.C. *et al.* (1977). Clinical Assessment of a Profession. Roman Catholic Clergyman. *Journal of Clinical Psychology 33*, 120-128.

Kerssemakers, J.H.N. (1989) *Psychotherapeuten en religie. Een verkennend onderzoek naar tegenoverdracht bij religieuze problematiek [Psychotherapists and Religion. An Exploratory Study of Countertransference with Respect to Religious Problems].* Nijmegen: Katholiek Studiecentrum.

Kirov, G., Kemp, P., Kirov, K. & David, A.S. (1998) Religious Faith after Psychotic Illness. *Psychopathology 31*, 234-245.

Koenig, H.G. (1990) Research on Religion and Mental Health in Later Life. A Review and Commentary. *Journal of Geriatric Psychiatry 23*, 23-53.

Koenig, H.G., Cohen, H.J., Blazer, D.G., Pieper, C., Meador, K.G., Shelp, F., Goli, V. & DiPasquale, B. (1992) Religious Coping and Depression Among Elderly, Hospitalized Medically Ill Men. *American Journal of Psychiatry 149*, 1693-1700.

Koenig, H.G., Larson, D.B. & Matthews, D.A. (1996) Religion and Psychotherapy with Older Adults. *Journal of Geriatric Psychiatry 29*, 155-184.

Koenig, H.G., Parkerson, G.R. Jr. & Meador, K.G. (1997) Religion Index for Psychiatric Research. *American Journal of Psychiatry 153*, 885-886.

Krause, N. & Tran, T.V. (1989) Stress and Religious Involvement among Elderly Black Adults. *Journal of Gerontology. Social Sciences 44*, 4-13.

Kurth, C.J. (1961) Psychiatric and Psychological Selection of Candidates for the Sisterhood. *Guild of Catholic Psychiatrists Bulletin 8*, 19-25.

Lans, van der J. (1981) *Volgelingen van de goeroe. Hedendaagse religieuze bewegingen in Nederland [Followers of the Guru. Present-Day Religious Movements in the Netherlands]*. Baarn: Ambo.

Lans, van der J., Pieper, J. & Uden, van M. (1993) Levensbeschouwing en geloof in de geestelijke gezondheidszorg. Een onderzoek onder Riagg-hulpverleners [Worldview and Faith in Mental Health Care. An Investigation among Riagg Staff]. *Psyche & Geloof 4*, 111-125.

Lazarus, R.S. & Folkman, S. (1984) *Stress, Appraisal, and Coping*. New York: Springer.

Lea, G. (1982) Religion, Mental Health and Clinical Issues. *Journal of Religion and Mental Health 21*, 336-351.

Leuba, J.H. (1896) A Study in the Psychology of Religious Phenomena. *American Journal of Psychology 7*, 309-385.

Lofland, J. & Stark, R. (1965) Becoming a World Saver. A Theory of Conversion to a Deviant Perspective. *American Sociological Review 30*, 862-874.

Luchtmeijer, G., Verbiest, K. & Wouters, I. (2001) *Spiritualiteit, een bepaling van het concept. Een zoektocht naar eenheid in de veelheid [Spirituality, a Conceptualisation. A Quest for Unity within Diversity]*. Unpublished manuscript, University of Louvain.

Lukken, G. (1988) *Geen leven zonder rituelen [No Life without Rituals]*. Baarn: Ambo.

Lukoff, D., Lu, F. & Turner, R. (1992) Toward a More Culturally Sensitive DSM-IV. Psychoreligious and Psychospiritual Problems. *The Journal of Nervous and Mental Disease 180*, 673-682.

Matthews, D.A., McCullough, M.E., Larson, D.B., Koenig, H.G., Swyers, J.P. & Greenwold Milano, M. (1998) Religious Commitment and Health Status. A Review of the Research and Implications for Family Medicine. *Archive for Family and Medicine 7*, 118-124.

Mead, G.H. (1934) *Mind, Self and Society*. Chicago: University of Chicago Press.

Meylink, W.D. & Gorsuch, R.L. (1988) Relationship between Clergy and Psychologists. The Empirical Data. *Journal of Psychology and Christianity 7*, 56-72.

Molenkamp, R. (1994) Depressief of troosteloos, een belangrijk onderscheid [Depressed or Disconsolate, an Important Distinction]. *Zin in Welzijn 5*, 2-5.

Morris, P.A. (1982) The Effect of Pilgrimage on Anxiety, Depression and Religious Attitude. *Psychological Medicine 12*, 291-294.

Nvagg. (1989). *Inventarisatie met betrekking tot cliënten van gereformeerde gezindte [Stock-Taking with Respect to Clients from the Reformed Denomination]*. Interne nota. Utrecht.

Nvagg. (1990). *Verslag onderzoek kwaliteitsbeleid Riagg's [Report on a Study of Riaggs' Policies regarding Quality]*. Utrecht.

Oosterwijk, J., Hoenkamp-Bisschops, A., Pieper, J., & Uden, van M.H.F. (1987) *Steun en ontmoeting. Een onderzoek onder bedevaartgangers naar Lourdes [Support and Encounter. A Study of Pilgrims to Lourdes]*. Heerlen: Universiteit voor Theologie en Pastoraat.

Paloutzian, R.F. (1983) *Invitation to the Psychology of Religion.* Glenview: Scott/Foresman.

Pargament, K.I. (1990) God Help Me. Toward a Theoretical Framework of Coping for the Psychology of Religion. *Research in the Social Scientific Study of Religion 2*, 195-224.

Pargament, K.I. (1997) *The Psychology of Religion and Coping. Theory, Research, Practice*. New York: The Guilford Press.

Pargament, K.I., Ensing, D.S., Falgout, K., Olsen, H., Reilly, B., Haitsma, van K. & Warren, R. (1990) God Help Me (I): Religious Coping Efforts as Predictors of the Outcomes to Significant Negative Life Events. *American Journal of Community Psychology 18*, 793-824.

Pargament, K.I., Kennell, J., Hathaway, W., Grevengoed, N., Newman, J. & Jones, W. (1988) Religion and the Problem-Solving Process. Three Styles of Coping. *Journal for the Scientific Study of Religion 27*, 90-104.

Pargament, K.I., Koenig, H.G. & Perez, L.M. (2000) The Many Methods of Religious Coping. Development and Initial Validation of the RCOPE. *Journal of Clinical Psychology 56/4*, 519-543.

Pargament, K.I., Olsen, H., Reilly, B., Falgout, K., Ensing, D.S. & Haitsma, van K. (1992). God Help Me (II): The Relationship of Religious Orientations to Religious Coping with Negative Life Events. *Journal for the Scientific Study of Religion 31*, 504-513.

Pargament, K.I., Smith, B.W., Koenig, H.G. & Perez, L.M. (1998) Patterns of Positive and Negative Religious Coping with Major Life Stressors. *Journal for the Scientific Study of Religion 37*, 710-724.

Pargament, K.I., Tarakeshwar, N., Ellison, C.G. & Wulff, K.M. (2001) Religious Coping among the Religious. The Relationships between Religious Coping and Well-Being in a National Sample of Presbyterian Clergy, Elders and Members. *Journal for the Scientific Study of Religion 40*, 497-513.

Pargament, K.I., Zinnbauer, B.J., Scott, A.B., Butter, E.M., Zerowin, J. & Stanik, P. (1998) Red Flags and Religious Coping. Identifying some Religious Warning Signs among People in Crisis. *Journal of Clinical Psychology 54*, 77-89.

Park, C.L. & Cohen, L.H. (1993) Religious and Non-Religious Coping with the Death of a Friend. *Cognitive Therapy and Research 17*, 561-577.

Parker, G.B. & Brown, L.B. (1982) Coping Behaviors that Mediate between Life Events and Depression. *Archives of General Psychiatry 39*, 1386-1391.

Pieper, J.Z.T. (1988) *God gezocht en gevonden? Een godsdienstpsychologisch onderzoek rond het kerkelijk huwelijk met pastoraaltheologische consequenties [God Searched and Found? Research in the Psychology of Religion regarding Church Weddings, with Pastoral Theological Consequences]*. Nijmegen: Dekker & van de Vegt.

Pieper, J.Z.T. (2004) Religious Resources of Psychiatric Inpatients. Religious Coping in Highly Religious Inpatients. *Mental Health, Religion and Culture 7/4*, 349-363.

Pieper, J.Z.T., Oosterwijk, J.W. & Uden, van M.H.F. (1988) Bedevaart: Steun en ontmoeting. Over de bedevaart naar Lourdes [Pilgrimage: Support and Encounter. On the Pilgrimage to Lourdes]. In: Uden, van M. & Post P. (eds.) *Christelijke bedevaarten. Op weg naar heil en heling [Christian Pilgrimage. On the Road to Salvation and Healing]*. Nijmegen: Dekker & van de Vegt, 159-170.

Pieper, J. & Uden, van M. (1991) De huidige Lourdesbedevaart. Motieven en effecten [Present-Day Pilgrimage to Lourdes. Motives and Effects]. In: Uden, van M. & Pieper, J. (eds.) *Bedevaart als volksreligieus ritueel. [Pilgrimage as a Popular Religious Ritual]*. Heerlen: UTP-teksten 16, 7-26.

Pieper, J.Z.T. & Uden, van M.H.F. (1993) *Ex-cliënten over de Riagg-OZL. Resultaten van een satisfactieonderzoek onder cliënten van wie de behandeling bij de Riagg-OZL te Heerlen in 1991 is afgesloten [Former Clients about the Riagg-OZL. Results of a Satisfaction Survey among Clients whose Treatment in the Riagg-OZL in*

Heerlen has been Completed in 1991]. Heerlen: Universiteit voor Theologie en Pastoraat.

Pieper, J.Z.T. & Uden, van M.H.F. (1993) *Ex-cliënten over de Riagg Zwolle. Resultaten van een satisfactieonderzoek onder cliënten van wie de behandeling bij de Riagg Zwolle in 1991 is afgesloten [Former Clients about the Riagg Zwolle. Results of a Satisfaction Survey among Clients whose Treatment in the Riagg Zwolle has been Completed in 1991]*. Heerlen: Universiteit voor Theologie en Pastoraat.

Pieper, J.Z.T. & Uden, van M.H.F. (1993) *Tevredenheidsonderzoek ouderen. Ex-cliënten van de afdeling ouderen over de Riagg-OZL [Satisfaction Survey among Elderly. Former Unit for Elderly Clients about the Riagg-OZL]*. Heerlen: OZL.

Pieper, J.Z.T., Uden, van M.H.F. (1996) Geloof en levensbeschouwing binnen de Riagg-hulpverlening. Ex-cliënten aan het woord [Faith and Worldview in Riagg Treatment. Former Clients' Views]. *Psyche & geloof 7*, 115-127.

Pieper, J.Z.T. & Uden, van M.H.F. (1996) Religion in Mental Healt Care. Patients' views. In: Verhagen, P.J. & Glas, G. (eds.) *Psyche and Faith. Beyond Professionalism*. Zoetermeer: Boekencentrum, 69-83.

Pieper, J.Z.T. & Uden, van M.H.F. (1997) *Geloof en levensbeschouwing binnen de Gliagg Dordrecht. Houdingen van therapeuten [Faith and Worldview in the Dordrecht Gliagg. Therapists' Attitudes]*. KUN-rapport: Heerlen.

Pieper, J.Z.T. & Uden, van M.H.F. (1997) *Geloof en levensbeschouwing binnen de Riagg's te Heerlen en Sittard. Houdingen van therapeuten [Faith and Worldview in the Heerlen and Sittard Riaggs. Therapists' Attitudes]*. KUN-rapport: Heerlen.

Pieper, J.Z.T., Uden, van M.H.F. (1998) Religieuze hulpverlening. Gliagg-therapeuten over geloof en levensbeschouwing [Religious Treatment. Gliagg Therapists' Views on Faith and Worldview]. In: Uden van M. & Pieper, J. (eds.). *Wat baat religie? Godsdienstpsychologen en godsdienstsociologen over het nut van religie [Religion to What Avail? Psychologists and Sociologists of Religion on the Benefits of Religion]*. Nijmegen: KSGV, 47-66.

Pieper, J.Z.T. & Uden, van M.H.F. (1998) Riagg-therapeuten over geloof en levensbeschouwing [Riagg Therapists' Views on Faith and Worldview]. In: Janssen, J., Uden, van M, & Ven, van der J. (eds.) *Schering en inslag. Opstellen over religie in de hedendaagse cultuur [Normal Practice. Essays on Religion in Present-Day Culture]*. Nijmegen: KSGV, 52-74.

Pieper, J.Z.T. & Uden, van M.H.F. (2001) *Geestelijke verzorging op De Fontein. Onderzoek onder cliënten van De Fontein naar hun geloof/levensbeschouwing en naar hun behoefte aan geestelijke verzorging [Pastoral Care at De Fontein. Research among Clients of De Fontein regarding their Faith/Worldview and their Need of Pastoral Care]*. Zeist (external report).

Ploeg, van der H.M., Defares, P.B. & Spielberger, C.D. (1980) *Handleiding bij de Zelf-Beoordelingsvragenlijst [Manual of the Self-Assessment Questionnaire]*. Lisse: Swets & Zeitlinger.

Pruyser, P.W. (1992) *Geloof en Verbeelding. Essays over levensbeschouwing en geestelijke gezondheid [Faith and Imagination. Essays on Worldview and Mental Health]*. Baarn: Ambo.

Raaijmakers, C. (1994) *Religie en hulpverlening. Een onderzoek naar de plaats van religie in de hulpverlening van de Riagg Groningen [Religion and Treatment. A Study of the Position of Religion in Riagg Groningen Treatment]* Groningen: Riagg Groningen.

Ragan, C., Newton Malony, H. & Beit-Hallahmi, B. (1980) Psychologists and religion. Professional Factors and Personal Belief. *Review of Religious Research 21*, 208-217.

Riagg en religie (landelijke werkgroep) (1991) *Beleidsnota 'Riagg en religie' [Riagg and Religion (National Task Force) (1991) Policy Document 'Riagg and Religion']*.

Richardson, J.T. (1985) Psychological and Psychiatric Studies of New Religions. In: Brown, L.B. *Advances in the Psychology of Religion*. Oxford: Pergamon, 209-223.

Rokeach, M. (1964) *The Three Christs of Ypsilanti*. New York: Knopf.

Schachtel, E.G. (1959) *Metamorphosis. On the Development of Affect, Perception and Memory*. New York: Basic Books.

Schaefer, C.A. & Gorsuch, R.L. (1992) Situational and Personal Variations in Religious Coping. *Journal for the Scientific Study of Religion 32*, 136-147.

Schilder, A. (1987) *Hulpeloos maar schuldig. Het verband tussen een gereformeerde paradox en depressie [Helpless Yet Guilty. The Connection between a Reformed Paradox and Depression]*. Kampen: Kok.

Schilder, A. (1991) Eigen over- of ongevoeligheden t.a.v. een christelijke levensbeschouwing [Our Own Hypersensitivities or Insensitivities towards a Christian Worldview]. In: Filius, R. & Visch, M. (eds.) *Zin in Welzijn. Over levensbeschouwing en professionaliteit in het welzijnswerk. [Meaning in Well-Being. About Worldview and Professionality in Welfare Work]*. Zwolle: Studiecentrum Welzijnswerk en Levensbeschouwing Windesheim, 41-49.

Schilder, A. (1991) Overtuiging, hulpverlening en verslaving [Belief, Help and Addiction]. *Zin in Welzijn 2*, 12-14.

Schilder, A., Schippers, A. (1990) *Religie in therapie [Religion within Therapy]*. Kampen: Kok.

Schuurman, I., Uden, van M.H.F. & Pieper, J.Z.T. (1999) Meer licht op levensbeschouwing in therapie. Een kwalitatief onderzoek naar levensbeschouwing onder Gliagg- en Riagg-therapeuten [More Light on Worldview in Therapy. A Qualitative Investigation among Gliagg and Riagg Therapists]. *Psyche en geloof 10*, 100-115.

Scott, E.L., Agresti, A.A. & Fitchett, G. (1998) Factor Analysis of the 'Spiritual Well-Being Scale' and its Clinical Utility with Psychiatric Inpatients. *Journal for the Scientific Study of Religion 37*, 314-321.

Spencer, J. (1975) The Mental Health of Jehovah's Witnesses. *British Journal of Psychiatry 126*, 556-559.

Spilka, B., Hood, R.W. & Gorsuch, R.L. (1985) *The Psychology of Religion. An Empirical Approach*. Englewood Cliffs, NY: Prentice Hall.

Starbuck, E.D. (1899) *The Psychology of Religion. An Empirical Study of the Growth of Religious Consciousness*. New York: Charles Scribner's Sons.

Stroeken, H. (1983) *Psychoanalyse, godsdienst en Boisen [Psychoanalysis, Religion and Boisen]*. Kampen: Kok.

Suls, J., David, J.P. & Harvey J.H. (1996) Personality and Coping. Three Generations of Research. *Journal of Personality 64/4*, 711-735.

Sundén, H. (1966) *Die Religion und die Rollen. Eine psychologische Untersuchung der Frömmigkeit [Religion and Roles. A Psychological Investigation of Piety]*. Berlin: Töpelmann.

Tepper, L., Rogers, S.A., Coleman, E.M. & Newton Malony, H. (2001) The Prevalence of Religious Coping among Persons with Persistent Mental Illness. *Psychiatric Services 52*, 660-665.

Uden, van M.H.F. (1985) *Religie in de crisis van de rouw. Een exploratief onderzoek d.m.v. diepte-interviews [Religion in the Crisis of*

Mourning. An Exploratory Study by Means of Depth Interviews].
Nijmegen: Dekker & van de Vegt.
Uden, van M. (1988) *Rouw, religie en ritueel [Mourning, Religion
and Ritual].* Baarn: Ambo.
Uden, van M.H.F. (1996) *Tussen zingeving en zinvinding. Onderweg
in de klinische godsdienstpsychologie [Between Imparting Meaning and Finding Meaning. En Route in the Clinical Psychology of
Religion].* Tilburg: Tilburg University Press.
Uden, van M.H.F. & Pieper, J.Z.T. (1990) Christian Pilgrimage. Mo-
tivational Structures and Ritual Functions. In: Heimbrock, H.G. &
Boudewijnse, H.B. (eds.) *Current Studies on Rituals. Perspectives
for the Psychology of Religion.* Amsterdam/Atlanta: Rodopi,
165-176.
Uden, van M.H.F. & Pieper, J.Z.T. (1996) *Religie in de geestelijke
gezondheidszorg [Religion in Mental Health Care].* Nijmegen:
KSGV.
Uden, van M.H.F. & Pieper, J.Z.T. (1998) Geloof en levensbeschou-
wing in de geestelijke gezondheidszorg [Faith and Worldview in
Mental Health Care]. In: Glas, G. (eds.). *Psychiatrie en religie. De
bijna verloren dimensie [Psychiatry and Religion. The Nearly-Lost
Dimension].* Nijmegen: KSGV, 75-97.
Uden, van M.H.F., Pieper, J.Z.T. (2000) Religion in Mental Health
Care. Psychotherapists' Views. *Archiv für Religionspsychologie
23,* 264-277.
Vellenga, S.J. (1992) *Zin, ziel, zorg. Over levensbeschouwing en gees-
telijke gezondheidszorg [Meaning, Soul, Care. On Worldview and
Mental Health Care].* Kampen: Kok.
Vergote, A. (1978) *Bekentenis en begeerte in de religie. Psychoanaly-
tische verkenning.* Antwerpen: De Nederlandsche Boekhandel.
[Vergote, A. (1987) *Guilt and Desire. Religious Attitudes and their
Pathological Derivations* [Transl. M.H. Wood], New Haven/Lon-
don: Yale University Press.]
Visch, M. (red.) (1991) *Leven beschouwen en hulp verlenen [World-
view and Helping].* Zwolle: SWL-Windesheim publ.
Vroon, P. (1978) *Stemmen van vroeger. Ontstaan en ontwikkeling van
het zelfbewustzijn [Voices of Yore. Origins and Development of
Self-Consciousness].* Baarn: Ambo.
Wal, van der J. (1991) *Principes en praxis van gereformeerde hulp-
verlening [Principles and Practice of Reformed Mental Health
Care].* Lezing op studiemiddag 'Riagg en geloof'. Tiel.

Wicks, R.J. (1985) My Values, your Values: my Defences, your Defences. Countertransference with clients of Different Religious Denominations. *Journal of Pastoral Counselling 20*, 47-52.

Wikström, O (1994) Psychotic (A-)Theism? The Cognitive Dilemmas of Two Psychiatric Episodes. In: Corveleyn, J. & Hutsebaut, D. (eds.) *Belief and Unbelief. Psychological Perspectives.* Amsterdam/Atlanta: Rodopi, 219-232.

Winnicott, D.W. (1971) *Playing and Reality.* New York: Tavistock.

Wong-McDonald, A. (2000) Surrender to God. An Additional Coping Style. *Journal of Psychology and Theology 28*, 149-162.

Worthington E.L. Jr. (1986) Religious counseling: A review of published empirical research. *Journal of Counseling and Development 64*, 421-431.

Worthington, E.L. Jr., Kurusu, T.A., McCullough, M.E. & Sandage, S.J. (1996) Empirical Research on Religion and Psychotherapeutic Processes and Outcomes: A 10-year Review and Research Prospectus. *Psychological Bulletin 119*, 448-478.

SUBJECT INDEX

ABOUT THE AUTHORS

Joseph Z.T. Pieper (1953) studied cultural psychology and psychology of religion at the Radboud University Nijmegen, the Netherlands. He received his PhD in psychology on a study on religious motivation for marrying in church. He works as an assistant professor in psychology of religion and pastoral psychology at the Department of Theology at Utrecht University and at the Catholic Theological University Utrecht, the Netherlands. Dr. Pieper has a long standing interest in research on religion and (mental) health and religious coping in mental health institutions. He also did research on the psychosocial effects of religious rituals, like pilgrimage, funerals and church weddings. He has been working on these subjects together with dr. Van Uden for almost two decades.

Marinus H.F. van Uden (1952) studied clinical psychology at the Radboud University Nijmegen, the Netherlands. He received his PhD in psychology on a study on the role of religion in grief. He was also trained as a clinical psychologist and psychotherapist (psychoanalysis and cognitive behaviour therapy) and maintains a psychotherapy practice in Heerlen, the Netherlands. He works as an associate professor in psychology of religion at the Department of Cultural and Personality Psychology at Radboud University Nijmegen. Since 1994 he was also appointed professor in clinical psychology of religion at the Theological Faculty of Tilburg University, the Netherlands. Dr. Van Uden has a long standing interest in research on religion, pilgrimage, individual rituals and mental health.

Printed in the United States
by Baker & Taylor Publisher Services